To
Jackie.

Hoody ...

I hope you find this inspirational.

Sylvia

x

Sylvia Hood

Contents

Introduction

This is the story of my son David's life, focusing in particular on his cancer diagnosis, his reaction and his two year battle. It is a mother's first-hand account of an experience no mother wants to go through, with surprisingly positive and uplifting elements, as well as the indescribable blow of losing a child.

Chapter one charts David's early life and chapter two deals more with the gifts and abilities he began to display as a teenager. For me chapter three is the most moving and shocking chapter, so much so that I can't easily read it now. It deals with David's anxious phone calls from a remote part of Southern Leyte, in the Philippines, saying 'You've got to get me home. This is not a knee injury. I'm dying!' He was right. Chapter four starts with the diagnosis of the tumour at the Royal Orthopaedic Hospital in Birmingham and then an insight into treatment at St James Hospital, Leeds. Chapter five gives the reader an insight into life on a Teenage Cancer Unit. Chapter six continues with the treatment at Leeds, Jimmy's, as it is more readily known. There is a focus on the awful chest drains and lung collapses, which kept David in bed for the first few months of treatment. This was a very difficult time for all of us, and many times we thought he was not going to live another day. Chapter seven explains the content of videos David made to tell his story. You can view these by googling David Hood and teenage cancer and going to JTV (Jimmy Teens T.V.) Positivity became David's lifeline and In chapter eight, I chart specific incidents where I was moved and sometimes bowled over by his response to very difficult situations. Chapter nine continues on this theme and shows how profoundly he touched people, young and old alike. Chapter ten begins to focus on the legacy of David's life and how people responded to his death. He was an inspirational young man, who touched the lives of many so positively.

Chapter 1
Early life

From pregnancy onwards our two children, Tom and David, were quite different. But as every mother would say, they were equally wonderful. Tom was born on August 1st 1987 and he was a very peaceful, easy to handle baby and toddler. David, on the other hand, did gymnastics in the womb and entered the world after a long labour on St Patrick's Day 1989. Ten days later he gave us a real scare when he stopped breathing and was rushed into hospital with Meningitis. Thankfully it was soon diagnosed and treated and within a week we were out of intensive care and back home with my husband John and Tom. After six months, he seemed to fully recover from all the antibiotics and it was hard to keep him satisfied on breast milk. He seemed to start then with a huge appetite for food and life.

Sport and the Christian faith dominated my life at this time. My first teaching job was at the prestigious Millfield School in Somerset[1977-81], where I was in charge of Hockey. I also coached Athletics, alongside teaching Mathematics and P.E. Following my working there for four years, I worked as an advisor to Christian Unions in the North East of England for the UCCF (Universities and Colleges Christian Fellowship). John had done a degree in Chemical Engineering and as he finished he decided not to pursue that career, and took off on the 'hippy' trail to India. When he returned home he took up a 'temporary' post at Longcroft Secondary School in Beverley as a science technician - a post that was to last the whole of his working life. Longcroft was the school where both of us had been as children and where we had vaguely known each other. It was also the school where I was later to return to teaching and Tom was to be a pupil. John and I got married and settled in Beverley in 1984.

Despite the fact that I was a workaholic, John and I had decided that it would be good for me to have a complete break from work whilst the children were young. We were both from 'good old fashioned Yorkshire families' where the woman stayed at home from when the children were born. John was an only child brought up in the village of Walkington and had been nurtured with a love of the countryside and nature. I was the youngest of four and brought up in the town of Beverley living a life full of sport and involvement in church activities. We wanted Tom and David to share some of the good experiences we had had. I can honestly say that I found the next five years some of the most varied, rewarding and creative years of my life.

Pre-school life: varied and full

I took the boys to Music Time, where I was soon helping to lead the actions in the nursery rhymes; Jack in the Box, which was gymnastics for pre-schoolers.; soft play, where they both loved clambering about; short tennis, with a lovely older lady doing the coaching, and Time Out, a church run playgroup and discussion session, as well as the usual coffee mornings and birthday parties, which I loved to host and lead.

It was at 'Time Out', held at Beverley Minster Parish rooms, that David's independent spirit first became evident to more than just me! He really had hit the terrible two's. I had been leading a challenging discussion on Christianity in a neighbouring room to the children's crèche and when I went to collect David from the crèche I sensed something was wrong. People were on edge. I asked someone what was wrong. 'Has no one told you?' they replied. 'David is missing and they're not sure how long he's been gone!' The person in charge of the crèche came up to me and burst out crying. 'Don't worry' I said, 'he'll turn up.'
'Where have you looked?' They told me they'd been all round the Minster and Sunday School rooms. 'I

3

would imagine he's gone into the town,' I said, and headed off up Highgate to the Wednesday market.

Within a hundred metres I found David, happy and smiling, playing with toys on the door step of the dentist. The receptionist had watched David following a couple to the zebra crossing adjacent to

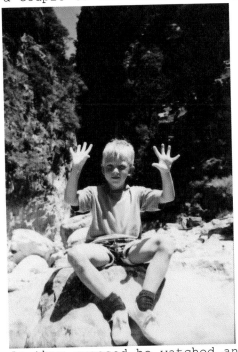

her door. As they crossed he watched and she thought they had left him. Then she realised he was on his own! She wisely took some toys outside to play with him where he could be seen. I was so grateful. I can't remember whether I was cross with him for wandering off or relieved to have found him. I know there were tears of joy and cuddles. Not so nine years later when he deliberately wandered off from the three of us in Pompeii one hot, sunny day! I think he got a well-deserved smack then!

Our first holiday abroad was when Tom was about five and Dave three. They really enjoyed swimming in a beautiful, turquoise bay in the south of Crete. They both thoroughly enjoyed building sandcastles and

4

playing in rock pools, catching crabs and the like. It was the first of many fantastic holidays abroad as a family.

Many happy days as youngsters were spent with two families in particular, who have remained excellent lifelong friends - the Delanoys and the Suttons. We had many memorable, themed birthday parties together and lovely dinner parties for the adults. Sue Banbury and in recent years, Mike and Sue's girls, joined this close knit group after returning to the UK from work in South America.

When talking about David recently all these friends commented on the exceptional amount of energy David had - an uncommon zest for life and a strong determination to pursue his dreams.

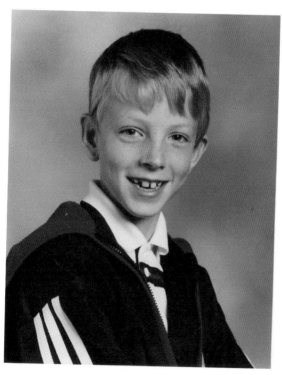

Claire Sutton recounted a good example of this:

I remember when we lived at Cherry Burton and David was about seven or eight. When it was time to leave, he said he wasn't ready to go home to bed and refused to get in the car. Sylvia suggested he ran home! A distance of about five miles which seemed a lot for his age. In independent spirit, he happily did this.

Sally wrote in his memory book of much earlier times of independently making his way home:

I struggled to keep hold of your hand as a little boy, because you wanted to be free and lead the way. Even then you had the confidence to know where you were going.

Sally and her youngest daughter, Fiona, recalled how when David was about four he walked home from their house on his own:

You came to collect him after school and he was being naughty so you told him to go and stand outside and wait until you were ready. When you went outside he had gone and you were unperturbed saying he will probably have walked home by himself.

How would he know the way, we thought? But sure enough, a short time later you phoned to say he was sat on the doorstep when you returned home.'

Independent Harry!

At church as a youngster he found it hard to sit still. Dave Hill (Junior) one of the church leader's son writes:

I have a lasting memory of holding a young, but very lively David between my legs to keep him still whilst Mum told Bible stories in Sunday School. FULL of life, lots of fun.

6

At the age of six he and Tom started to play chess seriously and they were soon in the regional team.

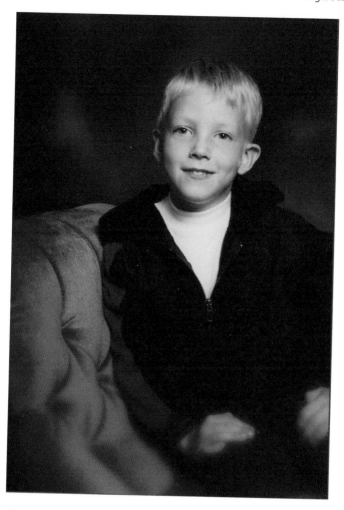

Chess soon disappeared into the background however and outside of school, where he loved Maths, tennis and music were the key activities. He played tennis most days of the week and thoroughly enjoyed learning the flute and piano. 'Ticking off' the grades in music exams seemed to satisfy him and by the age of ten he was keen to take his grade five theory, working out and being taught the mathematical 'tricks' for transposing music. A great love of music of many genres was something the boys shared. We were so chuffed that it included music of our era, the '70's, with the Beatles and Pink Floyd being high on their list of good music.

Chapter 2
From ten to teens

At the age of ten, David moved schools to Hymers College, a selective Independent School. With the financial implications of that decision, we simply couldn't afford to keep paying for tennis lessons and it was clear that without them Dave would not progress further than the fringes of county tennis. I therefore decided to introduce him to squash and he had lessons with a pupil I taught called George Bannister.

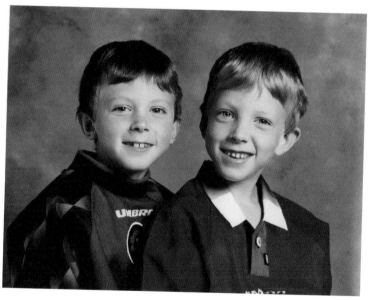

Tom and David

Together with another Hymers pupil, Bilail Iredale, we travelled to many tournaments in Yorkshire and they both were trained as part of the county squad. It was a fast, energetic game which suited David's temperament.

Memorable Times: from Bilail

SQUASH

- We used to play in David Lloyds. David was always a difficult player to play against. He could recognize his opponent's game very quickly. He was left handed (when most players were right handed) and he had an unorthodox double handed back hand, that was very difficult to read.
- We would be biting each other's heads off during a game, but as soon as it was over, we would shake hands and laugh all evening.
One time in particular that I remember, is when David and I were sat watching the England rugby match in David Lloyds, just after we had finished a game of squash and we were laughing so hard (due to David's jokes), that David choked on the famous cheeseburger he would always order after a squash game. I started to get worried, until he coughed the piece of burger out, which went flying across the room! Needless to say, we laughed even more!

ATHLETICS

- David was a naturally talented discus thrower! I remember him going on to represent North of England (and he barely ever trained!)
One time we were on the way to a regional finals athletics tournament and David and I were sat next to each other on the coach. It was a long journey so we had packed lunch. I took out a packet of cheese Doritos and offered one to David, to which he replied, "You shouldn't eat those, because they contain monosodium glutamate which can give you cancer!" Two years later David was diagnosed with cancer. That comment stuck in my head to this day!

10

At around the age of six Tom and Dave, as I mentioned earlier, began to learn and enjoy chess. John and I enjoyed the game and I decided to nurture this interest and sought out some chess coaching sessions. They were soon both in the regional team and playing tournaments with children and adults. It was amazing to go to conventions and see scores of youngsters motionless (well virtually) and speechless for much of the six matches, which could each last as long as an hour! If they lost quickly (or slowly) it was back to the 'rest'/play room to let off steam and regroup. David hated losing! Tom took it in his stride.

It was the same with short tennis, which David started when he was about four. He was so competitive and was soon in an elite squad and playing several times a week. Tom however, was more like John as regards sport, finding it tough and progress was slow.

Retrospectively, I think I was squeezed into the mould of the 'tennis mum' and I let David's drive and enthusiasm lead to 6.30 Sunday morning sessions! Free sessions for county hopefuls during school hours etc., he loved all of this highly focused coaching and by the age of eight had his first county representation. However, the price was the start of isolation at school from his football 'mates' as he had dropped football due to all the tennis matches which were necessary to climb higher up the ladder! There was only one other boy from Beverley who attended the coaching with David: Tom Davies. Today he is a very good professional tennis coach at my club in Beverley. All the others in the squad were from Hymers.

By the time David was ten everyone was telling me how unhappy he was - his flute teacher, his piano teacher, his tennis coach and other children's parents. David's behaviour at home took a downturn. He would slam doors, put 'keep out' notices on his little box room and scribble angry pictures. Then one day as he trudged home from school it all came out:

11

"I think I'll make everyone happy if I kill myself,"
he said. I couldn't believe it. Here was I, a mother
and a teacher, with a very unhappy child. "Why is it
that the more you achieve, the more you get picked
on?" he asked angrily. Then he burst out crying. I
fought back the tears and got him into the house as
soon as possible. His door was slammed! He let off
loads of steam and then we talked and planned.

He needed to move school I eventually decided after
several other very painful incidents occurred. But
where to? The neighbouring primary seemed a good
option but it was full. Eton offered to look at him
for a scholarship and I thought of Millfield but the
idea of sending him away from home when he was
vulnerable didn't seem right to John and me. We
decided Hymers College would be the best option,
even if it would break the bank for us. So, we
quietly arranged for him to sit the entrance exam
with no preparation and he was so chuffed when he
was offered a place. It was one of the best
decisions we have ever made as parents. He
flourished there. Within weeks he was coming top in
Maths tests and being held up, not bullied for doing
so. Also, the nickname 'Hoody' stuck.

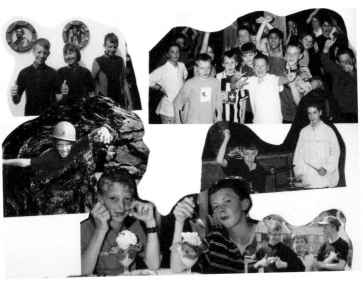

We thought Tom should have the same chances and so did others around us (who let us know their thoughts), but we couldn't afford two sets of fees. In any case, Tom was now happy at Longcroft and had his friends. In retrospect too, I think Tom would have hated Hymers and I think David would not have flourished so well at Longcroft. To parents who ask me to recommend state or private education, I always have to say that there are no easy answers. Some children will be happy in any school. Some thrive in one system, some in the other and some in neither.

The move to Hymers had financial implications for us and I gradually increased my teaching hours at Longcroft School, which had approached me to teach R.E. and P.E. It also meant that many of David's tennis lessons had to go. Squash replaced tennis and he was soon in the county squad with his good friend from Hymers, Bilail, who I mentioned earlier. Incidentally, Bilail is the grandson of the present owner of Hull City. Soon, the two of them also started doing some Athletics. I had been a county Javelin thrower in my day, but had never reached the international scene, with Tessa Sanderson and Fatima Whitbread ranking above me. My only claim to fame was winning the Yorkshire championships when they weren't there! David picked up Discus and Javelin quickly and was soon competing for the school and a local club.

By the age of 15 David looked and behaved like a man. (Well, most of the time that is!)

The three great loves of his life at this stage were athletics (especially throwing his discus), playing his flute and marine conservation.

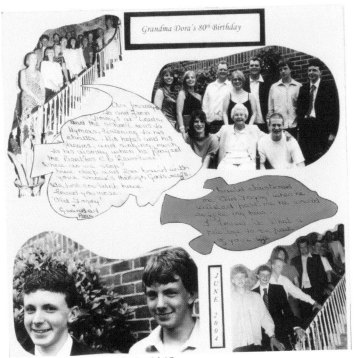

My mum's 80th. Tom 17, David 15.

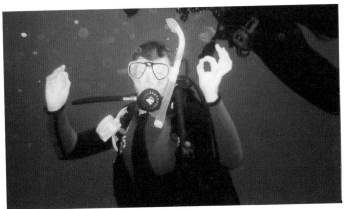

Diving. Dave taught me to dive.

At under 15 level he finished eighth in the country at the English Schools Championships and together with many other young people, he was encouraged to focus on the 2012 Olympics. He was throwing just under 40m. However, due to his growing interested in marine conservation, his throwing and multi-eventing took second place.

Academically he was very focused and during year 10 and 11 he began talking about trying to get into Cambridge to study Natural Sciences and eventually

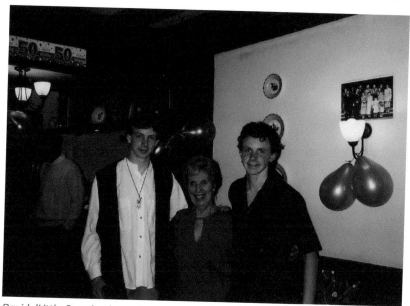

David, 'Little Grandma' and Tom

Marine Studies. Life was full and he was very happy. John and I seemed to be constant taxi drivers to one activity then another. Little Grandma helped too.

Marine Conservation becomes David's prime focus

One day his Physics teacher gave him a challenge which gave him a real focus in Year 10: a science project for a competition run by Hull University. He decided to look at the challenge of protecting the

world's marine environment. Amazingly he won the
individual prize: a two-week trip to Florida!

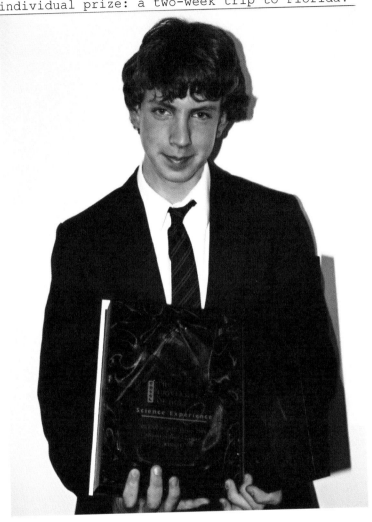

We were proud of him and he was so chuffed. So,
during the Easter holidays of 2005 he went on a
fabulous trip with five other students sponsored by
Hull University and six from Sunderland. They all
became very good friends. It seemed that David was
life and soul of the party on the trip and he was
instrumental in breaking down any barriers between
the two groups.

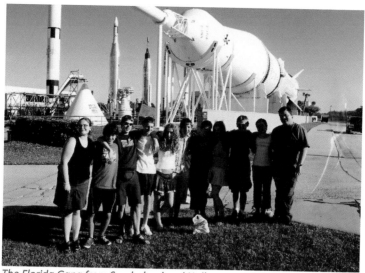

The Florida Gang from Sunderland and Hull

Following on from this fabulous trip, Dave decided to plan a marine focused trip with Coral Cay Conservation (CCC). As the Philippines seemed to have a great need to protect their environment, he asked if he could fundraise for a month-long trip there.

He worked so hard to raise the funds throughout Year 11, busking with his flute (he was now grade 8 standard) and mending computers, amongst other things. Anything to earn money, alongside GCSE exam preparations. Little did we know what was around the corner.

During the study leave for his GCSE exams he started getting a pain in his right thigh. Just before study leave he was hit by a football at the back of the thigh. The impact caused such pain that he said he was dead-legged and he fell to the floor, making him late back into registration. He started noticeably limping and by the June he was struggling to throw the Discus and put the shot in the County Athletics Championships. He withdrew from the competition sacrificing competing at the Nationals that summer and being more determined to put all his energies into his conservation trip in the Philippines.

17

Chapter 3
A mother's worst nightmare

"Mum, I'm seriously ill!"

These were not the words I wanted or expected to hear from David when he rang from his long anticipated trip to the Philippines. The person on the phone was my son David, also known as "Hoody."

"I can't eat. I can't sleep. I can't walk. I certainly can't dive. You've got to get me home."

What he said next drained the blood from my face.

"Mum, I think I'm dying."

This was my sixteen year old son. He had worked hard all year fundraising for the trip of a lifetime to join a marine conservation team based in a remote part of Southern Leyte in the Philippines. The journey from the UK to the base had taken three days. I therefore knew the practical implications of going to David's aid. Even if I made an immediate, impulsive response to travel, it would take half a week to get to him.

But David was clearly in distress.

"It's not a simple knee injury," he cried. "Mum, there's something seriously wrong and if you don't get me home I'm going to die. I'm sat outside on a grotty toilet with no seat. I'm trying not to wake anyone else but the pain is so bad I can't sleep."

I tried to remain calm and rational so as not to add to David's anxiety. "Describe the pain to me and the course it takes from your leg."

"It's so bad I think I am going mad! It starts in my leg and runs up to my hip then on to the base of my spine and up my back."

"That sounds like sciatica to me," I replied, trying to alleviate his anxiety.

"What's sciatica?"

"If you've been sat around for a number of days, as you were on the journey, your sciatic nerve, which runs up your leg and to your spine, can get trapped and cause intense pain."

"What shall I do?"

"Don't dive until we know what the problem is and keep mobile. Go snorkelling tomorrow and I'll phone you again and speak to Justin [the expedition leader] during the day and we'll take it from there."

"But the pain is so bad, mum. I can't think properly...I think I'm going mad!"

"David, I can't be with you and I can't be certain about what's wrong with you. Try what I have said. The best advice I can give you is to focus your mind on something else and pray. You said when you were eight-years old that you asked Jesus into your life and that you believe in God. So pray like you've never prayed before and God will be there with you and help you."

"I am trying to learn the Latin names of the fish and the coral," David groaned, "but it's hard because I can't sit up in the lectures. It's tough to concentrate because of the pain." David paused and then added, "I have been praying, and you know mum, God is closer than you could ever imagine!"

"I love you David," I replied as my eyes filled with tears.

"Love you too mum...speak to you tomorrow. Goodnight."

I tried not to panic and resolved to hope that my son would soon feel much better. But to my dismay things got worse. After several phone calls, David's acute pain and growing panic was becoming evident.

Boat Trip from Hell

"You've got to get me home." David repeated. "A nurse visits at times and injects me but the pain is so bad!"

It was time to act. I asked Justin to take David to the local doctor. This turned out to be a waste of time because he misdiagnosed David's condition as muscular-skeletal pain.

I then decided to contact the insurance company and ask for their advice.

"David needs an X-ray and medical attention," I insisted.

They implied that I was paranoid and over-reacting.

"In any case," they added, "the area he's in is too remote for us to get an X-ray. We will probably need to air-lift him to Cebu. However, if there's nothing wrong and it turns out to be a kneejerk reaction, you may end up paying a lot of money for this."

"What other options are there?" I asked.

"He could travel overnight by boat to Cebu and we could arrange for an X-ray there and then you can make plans to get him on a flight if necessary."

I phoned David and he agreed that this would be the safest (or, from the insurance company's point of view, the cheapest) option.

"I'll go with David to Cebu," Justin said.

How David made that journey I will never know. The pain must have been awful. He later told me how he had travelled in the early hours of the morning and had chosen to lie down in the bottom of the boat because of the pain. This turned out to be a nightmare because he kept getting kicked by others.

Having arrived at Cebu, Justin, wanting to make David's final day of the trip memorable, offered to take him to McDonalds. However, David later told me that even climbing the stairs required a momentous fight against the pain and that thinking about food turned his stomach. Eventually they arrived at a first class private hospital where the care was excellent.

About to Snap

A simple X-ray (which is what I had asked for repeatedly in England) showed that the femur of his right leg was about to snap in two. A huge growth had eaten it away and this, not a simple knee injury, was the cause of the abnormal swelling in the leg and the intense pain.

Much of what happened after that is a blur.

David's consultant sent us an email asking us to contact the hospital while decisions were taken as to what to do next. The hospital wanted to conduct an MRI scan. Sadly this took an eternity to complete because the pain was so intense David struggled to keep his leg still. The whole procedure consequently took much longer than expected.

When I eventually made contact with the consultant he expressed concern about putting David on a plane home because of the growth they had found on the femur.

The consultant was unsure anyway whether the growth was malignant. The pressing issue seemed to be whether or not the femur would break in two during the flight.

Just the thought of what David must have been going through sent me into a tailspin of turmoil. My son was too weak and sick to travel home. I was the other side of the world. It was crap and I was in shock.

It seemed that the trip of a lifetime was about to end in disaster. My baby was in agony and I, and to

21

a certain extent those around him, didn't really know what was wrong. What we did know didn't fill me with optimism.

After lots of phone calls and pleading emails from me, it was decided that Dave should be put on a plane with his leg in a brace and that he should be accompanied by a medical representative organised by the insurance company. Sadly, this person was never provided.

The next few days were filled with frenetic activity. It would take three days for Dave to travel home and he would land on August 1st, Tom's birthday.

We decided to move Tom's 18th birthday party celebrations so they could have their own space before David arrived home. I remember buying a marquee to fit between the house and the garage. This was to keep the lads (and of course the girls) outside while drinking and barbecuing.

I also decided to prepare all my R.E. work for the autumn term, anticipating David needing to be in hospital to have the growth examined.

That's about all I can remember.

We had no idea what was to hit us next.

The Weeping Doctor

The young man who was wheeled off the plane in Manchester on August 1st 2005, aged sixteen, was a shadow of the one we had waved off two weeks earlier. He had lost so much weight and his face was ashen with pain. Anguish is the only word I can think of to describe the look in his eyes. Thankfully there was some relief in seeing John and me. He just wanted to get to the privacy of our car and tell us about his ordeal. He also wanted to remove his leg brace.

Dave then just wanted to get home. So, home we went.

Much of that day was filled with hugs, phone calls and prayers. I was torn apart inwardly but tried to put on a brave face. I can't remember if I cried. I can remember that the hospital in Cebu had told us to phone our doctor and ask us to make plans for a chest X-ray the day after we got David home.

Chest X-ray? We thought. That's crazy. It's his leg not his chest that has a growth!

How wrong we were.

As the day progressed, David's agonising pain was clearly greater than he could bear and paracetamol didn't seem to touch it at all. By night time he was screaming in pain - and I mean screaming - and we didn't know what to do. We put him in our bed, trying our best to support the leg with pillows, icing the knee where the major swelling still was. But the pain did not abate. David was writhing on the bed. It reminded me of the agony I had seen my grandma suffer when I was a child. Gangrene was eating away her leg as she lay dying.

Agonising hours went by. Sleep was out of the question.

We began to catch a glimpse of the suffering David had endured by himself, the other side of the world. It made me feel sick, frightened, angry and utterly helpless.

Eventually, we decided to phone the doctor on call that night. It seemed ages before anyone arrived and we wondered what the neighbours must be thinking as they heard David's screams.

When the doctor arrived I briefly explained the whole scenario. He followed me up to the bedroom.

As soon as he saw David he started to cry.

I took him next door to console him.

"I'm sorry," he said. "I have a son about the same age. I have never seen anything like this."

"What can you do for him to quell the pain?"

"Nothing I can give will really touch that pain. He needs specialist care."

The doctor left and we were given a prescription for some painkillers to collect in the morning. He reminded us to go for a chest X-ray in the morning.

Nothing more was said.

I can't remember how John, Tom and I slept that night. We probably didn't.

David dozed at times, between the episodes of intense pain. It seemed that the type or the dose of medication was sadly lacking.

He looked so exhausted and frightened.

"The Big C"

Morning came and with it the challenge of moving David downstairs and into the car. We were supposed to have kept the leg brace on but he'd been in such discomfort with it that he insisted we remove it as soon as he had got into the car in Manchester. We suggested he ought to put it back on while we moved him from our bed to Hull Royal Infirmary.

It was on that day and in that hospital that cancer was first mentioned.

We took David down to the X-ray department, as instructed. Afterwards we gathered in a room full of staff. We were told that the growth on David's leg was cancer and that the cancer had spread to both the lungs.

We were all speechless.

They showed us the X-rays. It looked like a snowstorm had hit them.

We were now in a whirlwind of emotions. We were exhausted, running on adrenaline, worried, praying

24

continuously. It would be a miracle now if David managed to compete at the 2012 Olympics.

David was right: he was dying. In fact we were given the impression he might not live much longer. We weren't told much more. What we were given was instructions. Yes, not empathy or concern, but instructions. We were to go home and wait to be called to the Royal Orthopaedic Hospital in Birmingham. They had experts there who could diagnose what type of cancer it was, whether treatment would be useful, what approach, if any, might be effective.

We drove home feeling very inadequate about caring for David. Our lives had been turned upside down.

Our fit, healthy young son was now fighting for his life.

A Trip to the Deep

Back home from the hospital David initially didn't know how to respond. I didn't know what to say. How angry he must have been. Tom remembers one of us saying, "Throw something if you want! Throw something through the television if you have to!" David didn't throw anything. Instead he made plans.

"If I am going into hospital in about a week then I want to do something. Can I take my closest friends to The Deep? I'd like to go and see the fish and take my underwater camera and see if they will use it there as I've not used it in the Philippines."

I was soon organising this outing to Hull's celebrated aquarium and yet there was great concern surrounding the whole trip. As a teacher at Hymers College, as well as a parent, I felt it was my duty to inform the parents of David's friends and ask them if they wanted their child to be involved in the trip, or even visit David, especially since the prognosis might not be good. So I phoned them. Some were away, some at home. Their response was one of great shock at the news but they were all 100%

25

positive about wanting to visit and support David and the family.

Patrick and his dad Eugene were the first to visit. I was most grateful to Eugene for the time and advice he gave as a doctor. I remember well sitting at the bottom of our garden with him, whilst Patrick went upstairs to see David. It was a hot, sunny, summer's day and I found Eugene a really easy guy to talk to. "Increase the dosage of David's medication to a level that keeps the pain more at bay," he urged. Eugene explained that we may even need to give three times the dosage and he provided the reason for this. I loved his Irish accent, his sense of humour, his empathy and general manner. Dave really appreciated Patrick's visit too.

The visit to The Deep in Hull went ahead and the staff there really pulled out all the stops. They had arranged to loan a wheelchair with a leg extension, which turned out to be awkward to manoeuvre due to his long legs. They gave him a teddy bear (affectionately known in the family as "Blue Ted"), a book and other freebies.

Chapter 4
Birmingham

We drove to the Royal Orthopaedic Hospital unsure of what to expect. The staff were very welcoming and professional. They quickly realised that we had a very poorly boy on our hands and their first priority was to get the pain under control. This was not an easy task. Their deep concern about David's condition was evident and they communicated that he may only have three weeks to live without treatment. The storm hit us with all its force though when they said that treatment may be futile!! With such news, I found that one goes into shock and onto autopilot. Keeping this information away from David and comforting him and encouraging others to pray seemed to be the positive response. The prognosis was very poor.

We naturally wanted treatment and we wanted it to be started as soon as possible. However, as with many complex illnesses there was a certain protocol to follow and we were now in the hands of the medics there.

First, they needed to get the pain under control and they decided to run a line right down his leg to the source of his pain. Another line was put in his wrist and he was also given oral medication. It took three excellent doctors three days to get the pain under control and David was also given some control in all of this by having a device he could press to release pain relief straight into the tumour site. How he had coped in the Philippines we will never know and what would have happened if I hadn't moved his flight doesn't bear thinking about.

The support from Beverley Baptist Church, where we were members, was first rate. Newsletters were sent out to inform people how things were progressing with David's treatment and what things needed to be prayed for. This took a lot of pressure from us and the whole family drew great strength and encouragement from this. I still have copies of all the e-mails. The following is an extract from one dated August 9th 2005:

David was initially admitted into quite a large, busy ward, which Sylvia was concerned would make it difficult for him to rest. In fact, this afternoon David has not been at all well, so he was moved into an individual room, which is better. He has not eaten much and is clearly in a lot of pain from his leg.

Once in his room, David suffered what seems to be an allergic reaction to the bedding, so had the discomfort of an itchy rash in addition to everything else. He now has fresh bedding and a pressure mattress, and he is now more comfortable. He has a morphine drip which he can control himself, to ease the pain. Please pray for a good night's sleep for him. John will be sleeping in the room with him tonight, while Sylvia has a room in the nurses' home.

We do need to pray for God's peace for David; being in the hospital environment, with lots of very ill children and hearing the medical staff's reaction to his illness, has made him become increasingly more aware of the severity of his situation - it is very frightening for him.

This afternoon Dave has had a CT scan and X-rays, to assess whether there is any spread from his leg to other parts of his body (particularly the lungs). The results are not available today - they hope to get them tomorrow. Please pray that these will be clear.

On Tuesday David will have a full bone imaging scan, and probably a biopsy on Wednesday before coming home. The result of the biopsy will take 7 days to come. At the moment Sylvia is not sure that David would be well enough to travel home in the car: pray that he will be more comfortable by Wednesday. They have been told that follow up treatment (i.e. chemotherapy) would probably be at Jimmy's in Leeds, which is at least less far to travel. However, if surgery is needed, this would mean more visits to Birmingham."

In talking with the staff the awful, gruesome way forward was becoming clear. The best case scenario was for the tumour to be identified quickly and then for chemotherapy to be started as soon as possible. If successful in shrinking the primary tumour (the one on the leg) and the secondary's (the ones on the lungs and anywhere else) then we would be sent back to Birmingham from Jimmy's to have the leg amputated or if possible rebuilt. Contemplating all of this and having David involved in discussions in such a poorly state was soul destroying. The storm was buffeting us and we were working hard not to fall over.

Sleep was intermittent and troubled for all of us. David especially. When he did sleep he began to have nightmares due to the effects of the morphine. He said this was one of the worst aspects of the treatment there.

Church email update, Tuesday August 9th:

It has been a long day for David. He is eating very little and has been suffering from sickness. His pain relief has been interrupted by having to go to another hospital today for more tests.

There is still no definite feedback about the results of the scans and x-rays, because David and Sylvia have been at another hospital for much of the day, and haven't been able to talk to the consultant, who is busy in theatre etc. Continue to pray that the feedback from the scans will bring good news.

Pain is still a problem. The nurses have tried to put David on oral medication, in preparation for coming home, but his upset stomach is making this impossible, and he is now back on the morphine drip. Pray that David's stomach will settle so he can eat and have oral medication.

Sleeping arrangements have been working o.k. John has been sleeping in David's room, and then getting rest during the day while Sylvia is with David.

Do give thanks for wonderful support from medical and other staff. There appears to be plenty of support available for when the family comes home, including occupational therapists to look at adaptations needed at home.

David is due to have a biopsy tomorrow (Wednesday) and then should be coming home, if he is well enough. He is certainly not up to travelling by car at the moment, and would probably need an ambulance. Pray that his condition will improve for the journey home.

Longer term treatment plans are still dependent on the outcome of tests and the biopsy, as the medical team need to know exactly what kind of tumour they are dealing with.

It was excellent to have 20 people gathered together on Monday evening to pray for David and the family. Members of the Hood's family, good friends of many years, friends from several churches, and school friends of David's met together. We prayed that God will miraculously intervene and bring healing and restoration to David.

It was like being spun by a tornado. How to support David was our primary concern but we were also concerned to keep in touch with Tom, who was at home by himself. We had planned to go away to France that summer with our closest friends: Claire and Richard Sutton and Sally and Alan Delanoy and others. We cancelled our ferry tickets and between them our

30

lovely friends made arrangements for Tom still to go with them. It was a great distraction for Tom because most of the children going were Tom's age: Hannah, Josh, Evie, Emma, Fiona and others. We were so grateful to them helping us out in this way and their faithful support has continued right to the present day. They have been amazingly loyal and kind.

The only other thing I can remember from Birmingham was buying some warm pyjamas as the room I was staying in was so cold.

Chapter 5
St James' Hospital, Leeds (Jimmy's)

There were delays in getting David moved to Leeds due to a shortage of beds, so I drove home to Beverley for the weekend to be with Tom. Just before David had gone to the Philippines, John and I had gone on holiday to help my body recover from being ill for the first time in my life, and experiencing serious post viral fatigue. I could feel the aching in my muscles and the numbness in my feet returning as I drove north. In fact, as I reached the M1, I was finding it increasingly difficult to concentrate and I couldn't feel the accelerator. It was as if I had platform shoes on my feet, so I decided to stop for a coffee.

I remember meeting a family from Hymers who knew David well from the athletics team. I was, I suppose, in shock and so were they as I told them the news. It was hard fighting the tears back. This was another example of 'trying' to cope as a mother and a teacher.

It was good to be back home in my own bed for a short time, to catch up with Tom and make plans for him to go to France with my friends. Naturally, John, David and I were sad that we were not going as well. It was also good to see my friends from church and elsewhere and of course my mum and John's parents. The church e-mail was great for keeping people in touch and took some weight of us. It recounts the start of a pattern of travelling between Beverley and Leeds and John and I trying to spend time together with David, time trying to get some rest and for me time starting to prepare for the hockey pre-season and the start of an autumn term with no holiday. Far from it. It was a nightmare!

Church email update, August 16th:

> Tomorrow David will be having a small operation to have a central line fitted; he has also been having blood tests to make sure he is OK to start chemotherapy. The results of the biopsy etc. are back, and the tumour has been identified as osteosarcoma; this means that treatment can get going, although the earliest it will start would probably be Friday this week. Pray that the treatment will be effective and that any side effects will be minimal.
>
> The family has decided that John will be the main carer while David is having treatment in Leeds. John is visiting the GP tomorrow (Wednesday) morning to ask about being signed off work, which he was advised to do by the support staff in Birmingham. Pray that this will not be problematic. John will then travel back to Leeds tomorrow, and Sylvia will return for a while."

Visiting and living on ward 10T was a shock to the system itself. At the teenage end there was a four bed unit and two individual rooms. The younger children's ward was at the other end. I found it hard fighting the tears back as I saw babies and toddlers with Nasal Gastric (NG) tubes and main lines for chemo. Nonetheless, the whole atmosphere though was generally very positive, in spite of all the pain. The staff were all loving and professional.

The start of chemo for David had to be delayed in order to give him chance to discuss the possibility of sperm banking. He was a very sick boy. The leg was grossly swollen, he was struggling to eat and his future was uncertain. Because of the spread of the cancer to the lungs we were told that even with a year of chemo and operations, he still only had a 10% chance of surviving (David did not know this).

However, together we talked about the practicalities of sperm banking and frustratingly he had to go by wheelchair to another part of the hospital for counselling on this issue. Surprisingly he managed to masturbate and produce sperm in his condition, but he was glad to secure a future for himself as a parent should the chemo rob him of his fertility. I never thought he would have to contemplate such things at the age of 16.

After some discussion as to the pros and cons of treatment, chemo started, and so did the constant support with urine bottles, bed-pans, sick pans etc. but thankfully right at the beginning of treatment David did manage to get the odd day at home.

Church email update:

"Dear Friends

We: thought you'd appreciate a brief update on David Hood. Monica spoke to Sylvia this evening, and David is back home between chemotherapy treatments, probably for a brief time. This is a crucial period in his treatment and we need to pray that he will not catch any infections while his resistance is low. David is tired from the taxi journey home from Leeds after his exhausting hospital stay and presently feels weak and sick from the side effects, but he continues to show a brave and positive spirit. John and Sylvia are also understandably exhausted and overwhelmed with the whole situation, so let's pray for them too.

You'll be delighted to know that David's GCSE results were very good: 5A*'s, 4A's and a B. His school have agreed that if necessary he can take his A levels over a 3 year period." Two days later David had to be taken back to hospital with an unacceptably high temperature."

Two memorable highlights on the ward for David in particular, and us, were the Jolly Trolley and the visits of Dave Pettit: the parent of a child who had recovered somewhat and during his stay on the ward he became a Christian, through a vicar who lost his son. Nurse Jolly came round regularly with a smile and a sweet trolley for all the children and Dave

Pettit visited the ward once a week to talk to and pray with any patient or parent who wanted to. David really looked forward to Dave's visits and they would talk and pray together. Prayer became increasingly a natural part of David's life and a coping mechanism. I remember him once saying 'Pray when you're in pain. It's not the first thing that comes into your mind but it works to get rid of the pain.'

Dave Pettit had spent time on the ward himself with his son Harvey. During this time, he had become aware of God in a real way and with the help of a friend called Steve Redman, he had become a Christian. I am still in touch with Dave and sadly his son had a relapse this year and was re-admitted to Leeds for treatment. We spoke honestly together of cancer. I recalled how one day on the ward as I came back to the parents room after visiting a patient in whom the cancer had gone up to the brain, which was causing him to have fits and go blind, I said, 'it's crap'. To which another parents responded 'I didn't think you would use that word as a Christian! It's not just crap; it's crap, crap and more crap and when I get out of here I am going to preach a sermon on crap, crap and more crap and how in David's words your family, friends and having a faith get you through.'

Of cancer Dave used the word sh*t (or muck! He is an agronomist) and said 'sh*t is extremely valuable and leads to the most fruitful growth.' Of David he said 'He had a humility, a peace and a serenity that was tangible.'

Church email update 2nd September 2005:

> Sylvia phoned us last night to update us on David's condition. They had a long conversation with David's consultant at the hospital, where he has been given his own room, at least at present. David is in more pain with his leg; the lower leg is swollen as well as the upper leg, which prevents him from getting up, and his chest is painful. The consultant said this isn't necessarily a bad

35

sign and may indicate that the tumour is aggravated by the chemotherapy and may in fact be decreasing in size. He cannot be certain about this. The consultant was encouraging overall. He said David has coped marvellously with the feeding tube they have inserted, and they will increase the calorific intake so as to provide the nourishment he needs.

David is bearing up as much as he can. He told the consultant: 'I had such a perfect life before this, and now I can't do anything for myself.'

Church email update, September 8th

David had a brief time of respite at home after a tiring journey on Monday evening, when he enjoyed seeing some of his friends. He went back to hospital in Leeds on Tuesday evening and yesterday (Wednesday) he embarked on more chemotherapy - still part of round one. Today he will receive an antidote to protect his kidneys, and tomorrow he'll undergo a batch of test to check his blood quality etc. If all goes well and he's strong enough, he may be allowed back home for the weekend for a few more days before starting another dose of chemo.

The swelling is still very much in evidence and is putting pressure on the lower leg, ankle and foot. This is restricting the circulation somewhat and is very painful. Please pray that this will decrease. He is also now beginning to lose his hair, a temporary side effect of the chemotherapy. David is coping well with the feeding tube and getting nourishment as well as managing to eat small amounts himself. His temperature is still raised, but stable. The medical team think this may be due to the intense heat in the area of the tumour."

September 13th (the day before my 50th!)

David has now completed round one of his chemotherapy treatment, and is undergoing preparations for round two - a major onslaught due to start on Wednesday of this week. On Monday he received a blood transfusion and today (Tuesday) he receives hydration treatment to build him up for the chemo. He is expected to feel nauseous with this next round, so please pray about this, especially as he still has the feeding tube in place.

He may have the morphine line in his leg removed, as this may be causing the infection and raised temperature he still suffers from. It will also allow the hospital to check his level of pain at this time, and it may help his mobility. He will probably be put onto a more general morphine treatment subsequently.

David is on regular antibiotics, but they still haven't found the source of his infection. His high temperature may come from high activity in the tumour caused by the chemo. The overall circumference of his thigh has decreased by 4.5 centimetres, and the swelling in his lower leg and foot has gone down somewhat. This is encouraging, so keep praying, but it is not clear yet if this is linked to the tumour."

Keeping focused by producing video diaries

As he was so sick David decided to defer his A level studies and therefore when he was well enough he joined in with some of the activities on the ward. There was a parents' quiet room and a day room for parents and children where regular craft activities took place. Patients were also encouraged to tell the story of their battle with cancer, to help them come to terms with it and to inform and help others. David produced four videos in all, which can be viewed on www.jimmyteenstv.com - type David Hood into the search engine. The first one was largely filmed during the first four months of treatment,

37

the second when he was nearing the end of the first year of treatment, the third was with Marc Woods at the 'Find Your Sense of Tumour' conference in 2007 and the final one was filmed by the BBC largely, the

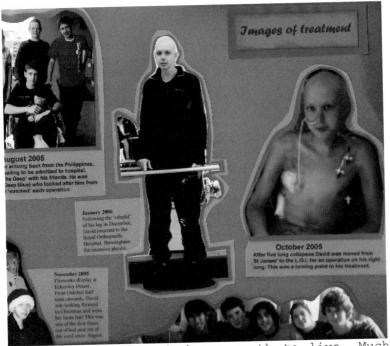

Images of treatment

August 2005
[...] arriving back from the Philippines, waiting to be admitted to hospital. [...] Deep' with his friends. He was [...] Blue) who looked after him from [...] 'watched' each operation.

January 2006
Following the 'rebuild' of his leg in December, David returned to the Royal Orthopaedic Hospital, Birmingham for intensive physio.

November 2005
Fireworks display at Eckersley House. From October half term onwards, David was looking forward to Christmas and wore his Santa hat! This was one of the first times out of bed and out of the ward since August.

October 2005
After five lung collapses David was moved from St James' to the L.G.I. for an operation on his right lung. This was a turning point in his treatment.

day he was told he had one month to live. Much of the fourth one is paralleled on the BBC news site and can be seen by again typing David Hood and teenage cancer into the search engine.

In David Hood part 1 he aims to give practical advice to other teenagers on chemo:

> You really need to get on top of your anti-sickness as soon as you're on it and drink lots so that you get rid of it quicker than usual and don't expect to do much while you're on it 'cos it takes everything out of yeh.

> I didn't react very well at the start of my chemo, being very ill and only having three short days at home with three months in hospital (tied to a wall with a chest drain).

You can't really eat your favourite things. First of all you have to take stuff out of your diet, like natural yogurt and seeing as I lost so much weight, they put me on this tube down the nose (naso-gastric tube) and it stops you eating things like bread, which is really quite annoying, well because bread's quite a big part of your diet, and in the end there's very little you can end up eating. You see, your favourite foods you may not like any more…it certainly happened to me - meat and potato pie: I tried it and it tasted just like plasticine. It's quite annoying really.

The chemo did its job though. It killed and made the tumours shrink very quickly. The trouble was though that it ripped holes in my lungs and caused many lung collapses.

The tumours are responding. They're shrinking. Some of them are quite big and basically as they've shrunk they've left holes around them and then the air can escape. It can happen either straight away or slowly. But if it happens straight away you feel as if you are going to die. You're in a lot of pain and you sometimes might start coughing and choking and being desperate for breath, even though your stats are fine, which is quite a weird experience."

In order to deal with the collapse of the lungs which the holes caused, David had to have many chest drains. If you will forgive the pun, these were draining for all of us! It was frightening to see him fighting for his breath and then having something akin to a metal barbeque skewer inserted between the ribs into the chest wall and then a plastic tube put down which attached him to a chest drain and inevitably a wall. He found the drains very frustrating as they prevented him from getting out of bed easily and prevented him from going home. As he said, 'the trouble with this chest drain is they can't let me home 'cos it's too much of a risk.'

39

I remember that on Bonfire night he was given a portable chest drain to enable him to have a break from the ward and go outside to watch the fireworks. Having lost all his hair, he wore his much loved Santa hat and he then wore it from then on, focusing on trying to get so much better so that he could get home for Christmas.

Another awfully memorable occasion was when he was in the side room (having been very sick again). He was attached to the wall with a painful chest drain, was being sick due to chemo., having diarrhoea again due to chemo and was holding an intense conversation with the consultant, Ian Lewis, as to how to prepare himself for the possibility of losing his leg! I marvelled at his composure and mental focus amidst so much distraction and pain.

In the video David Hood part 1 he asks his dad to interview him during this time and gives the following practical advice for anyone on similar treatment to him:

1. If you ever have an N.G. tube, remember to keep really relaxed and take sips of water regularly. I had to have about 16 of them in. The first one was a nightmare and took an hour to get down, but then I realised that if you try and sleep during it, it goes down really quickly.

2. Another piece of advice is if you can't take a shower or bath, keep yourself clean, especially your private parts as they are at risk of infection.

3. Keep positive - time seems to fly a lot quicker when you're positive. And keep your friends and family close as that helps as well. Friends will help you get through this and when they visit it seems to go a lot quicker.

4. Having a religion (or faith) is also a good thing. I found it hard in the Philippines as I started to go quite mad and I started talking to myself. But the fact that I had a faith gave

me someone to talk to. It helps a lot during the times of pain and suffering, there's always someone to turn to who can help you.

5. When you have a methatrexate chemo., the best bet is to drink as much as you can and piss as much as you can, as that gets it out of your system a lot quicker and that means you can get home, which is the best option for everyone.

6. When you find your hair starts to fall out, I would say your best bet is to shave it all off, as you will find you're spending a lot of time in hospital and having long hair isn't the best option as it gets dirty very quickly.

7. You might also find it helpful if one person does a weekly newsletter to update everyone as to how you're doing with your treatment as you don't have enough time to tell everyone yourself.

8. There are many charities that help people with cancer. One of them is the Robert Ogden Trust and they give free massages to those who ask for them. I find these very useful as they relax you and it makes you feel better.

Especially when he couldn't get out of bed, David looked forward to the hand, scalp and foot massages and he built up positive relationships with the staff. One commented as to how much she loved to massage his size 13 feet and how she 'saw' angels above his head and experienced a peace that seemed to emanate from him.

When he was terminal a lovely charity called the Willow Foundation gave David money for a 'special day'. He chose to spend it with his close friend Mady at a local spa having massages and other relaxing treatments.

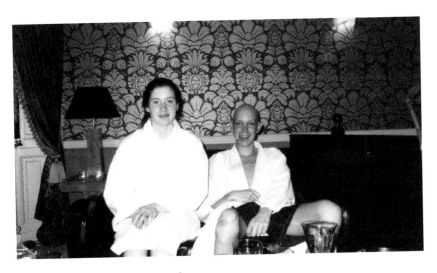

Mady and David relax at Sessions Spa

I was encouraged to join them by the charity. We had a super day at Sessions, where the staff were excellent. Lunch was also provided. The Willow Foundation is a national charity established in 1999 by the Arsenal footballer and BBC sports commentator Bob Wilson and his wife Megs as a lasting memorial to their daughter, Anna, who died of cancer aged 31.

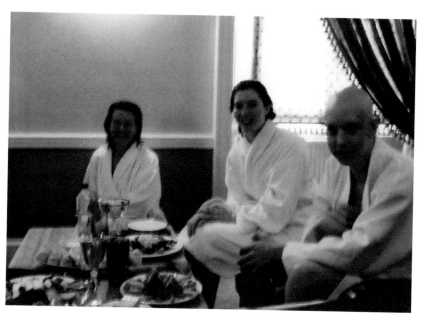

A healthy lunch

Two people who commented on his video, David Hood
part 1 say:

"I have just watched David's film and I think it
needs to be said what an amazing person he is. 18
years old yet extremely wise and intelligent. I am
completely blown away by David's positive attitude.
Wow! What an inspirational person. (Sharon Graves, 6
years ago)"

"Yeh, David was a smashing lad. I had the complete
honour of knowing him. His life has changed my life.
I view it now from a different spectrum. Miss you
bro'. (Carl Sage, 5 years ago)"

Chapter 6
The blessed lungs!

Church email update, October 16th

>There was a slight complication this weekend with David's tube which had been inserted to help re-inflate his right lung. A relatively junior doctor removed the tube last night, and for whatever reason the removal and stitching up took too long. The process went somewhat less well than it should have done, causing David a lot of pain and leading to some air enter the cavity at the side of his lung. Another consultant is to decide if David will need to have the tube reinserted. Understandably John and Sylvia were quite upset about this, but Sylvia reported this afternoon that David was more settled now and they feel more confident about the doctors supervising his treatment. We need to keep praying for the medics to have exceptional wisdom in all of this - they are as human as the rest of us!

>John spends every night sleeping on a fold-up bed next to David, and he is involved in caring for David's every need. He eats with David and sits with him during the day. I told him today he is a hero, but I think John would see this as normal for a Dad with his son. May God bless him and Sylvia with a peace that passes all human understanding.

Church email update, October 22nd

>This has been a week on many emotions for David and his family. Following the scan this week, they said that the tumours on the lungs were smaller, but there is a tendency for the lung to adhere to the chest wall, causing repeated problems. This weekend they will do more x-rays, and they will put a clamp on the

tube in his lung to see if he can do without it. If it is okay they will try removing it again; if not they will consider surgery.

For the first time David raised the question last weekend with the consultant whether his leg might need to be amputated if things didn't improve. The MRI scan showed very encouragingly that the tumour on his leg had only pushed aside the nerves and blood vessels, and had not eaten into them or surrounded them. This would make eventual surgery much easier. The consultant said he was happy with the progress David is making.

This young man is bravely fighting a battle that most of us couldn't contemplate. Let's keep asking God to provide all the strength he needs and more besides.

I was so touched as a mother that David's concern about losing his leg was not how would he be able to take part in all his sport, but how would he be able to walk in the Lake District with Tom with only one leg! Tom and David were so different but loved each other and supported each other.

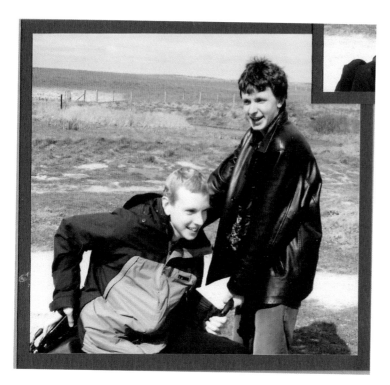

Tom and David

Now that Tom was a student in Leeds, he would visit the ward regularly. David would really look forward to him coming on a Friday night when he had more time, and they would spend time together listening to music, watching videos and chatting like any two teenagers but the whole environment, being so close to death of young people, wasn't what you would want your 16 and 18 year old to experience.

While the boys enjoyed time together, to help Tom, we would wash all his clothes on the ward or at Eckersley House.

Tom's support for David was first rate. When David was first diagnosed, whilst many were saying "why David?", as if he should be immune to the struggles and pain of this world, "Why not David?" said Tom. He can cope. And cope he did with the whole agonising situation.

24th November, Glynn [one of our best friends and a church leader co-ordinating contacts, prayer and news] writes:

> This is the best news we've been able to write so far! Really good news!
>
> David had his operation yesterday and it was a great success. The surgeons removed the tumour on his thigh and replaced the damaged femur with a titanium implant, so he woke up from the four hour operation with both legs intact! In a couple of days they expect him to stand up, then he'll need to get used to walking again, climbing stairs and being fully mobile.
>
> Also, the result from the biopsy on the tissue they removed from the lung a couple of weeks ago showed that the residue from the tumours was dead. So the chemotherapy has worked.
>
> John and Sylvia were delighted, and we all have good reason to be grateful to God and to be thankful for the skill and care of the medical staff who have worked with David.
>
> We haven't reached the end of this journey yet- in a couple of weeks David will undergo more chemotherapy, so let's keep praying for total healing, and for David to be strong enough to see it through.
>
> Nehemiah 8 v 10 says: "The joy that the Lord gives will make you strong."

This was indeed a more joyful time and after four months more or less solidly in hospital, David was focusing on being able to climb a flight of stairs (the bench mark for being allowed home) and looking forward to seeing family and friends again.

Within a week, he had pushed himself to climb a flight of stairs and through water and land-based physiotherapy he was learning to walk again! The Church email again explains:

> "David was out until midnight visiting with friends last night! That's quite a step forward from where he was not too long ago...
>
> We saw him this afternoon at home, and it was great to see him looking animated, happy to talk to us and the school friends who were visiting him, and his face looks so much more full and healthy. His friends took him out for a walk in the wheelchair, but he got up and walked with crutches in the house and he is looking forward to going swimming as part of his physiotherapy. He is eating three meals a day, and he's enjoying plenty of his favourite drink- milk! There's a lot to be thankful for.
>
> We saw pictures of the operation, which David had asked for. When they removed the tumour, it came out as part of a package containing much of the femur and surrounding muscles, and it was the size of a rugby ball!! They then put together a titanium rod to replace the femur, attaching it to the upper thigh bone and the lower knee joint. This is the wonder of modern surgery and a reason to give thanks for the NHS."

People showed their kindness through visits, cards, letters and we received mail - some from people we didn't know:

> "When I (Duncan, a friend from tennis) first heard about David's condition, I was very moved to hear of somebody so young being laid low by cancer. You always feel a bit helpless when you can't do anything to help apart from prayer and to offer encouraging words of support. But then I heard from a mutual friend of his mother's (Kate) that one of his favourite bands was Pink Floyd and my ears pricked up. Through a couple of meetings

backstage at gigs and at the Edinburgh fringe I had made the acquaintance of Guy Pratt, who was not only the part time bass player of Pink Floyd but also married to Gala Wright, the daughter of one of Pink Floyd's original members Richard Wright. I sent Guy Pratt an e-mail explaining David's situation and asking him if he could possibly get Richard to write a personal note to David to offer him encouragement and support. The note duly arrived and I took it to St James' Hospital in Leeds where David was at the time. I seem to remember him understandably being a bit surprised by my visit but his eyes lit up when he read the letter.

There is the theory of 'six degrees of separation' which puts forward the notion that we are all connected, so that everyone is six or fewer steps away by way of introduction from any other person in the world, so that a chain of contact can be created to connect any two people in a maximum of six steps. Here it was in action a chain of six people..."

David->Sylvia (His Mother)->Kate->Duncan(Me)->Guy Pratt->Richard Wright.

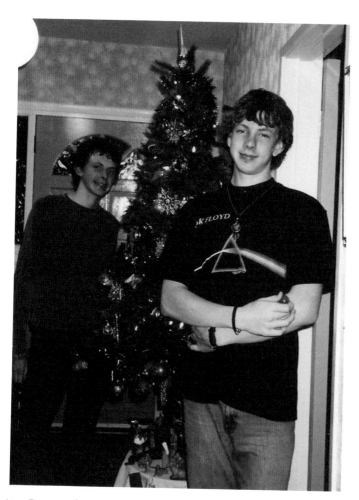

Hi David

I hear you are a great fan of our music
and I hope it has been a comfort for you.
I know you are very soon having an operation
and I want you to know my thoughts are with
you and I am sure all will go well.
Let me know how it went

Yours

Richard Wright   ("Pink Floyd")

Chapter 7
Positive responses which marked David out

How we respond to the great challenges of life, either good or bad can speak volumes to others. Throughout his life, but especially throughout the two years of a chronic and eventually terminal illness, David had extremely positive responses that those around him marvelled at and commented on many occasions. It is probably for that reason that ten years down the line from his passing, that I feel compelled to write on aspects of his life and especially about how he faced the trials of cancer and eventually how he faced death.

At the Service of Celebration of David's life, John Morris, David's Head Teacher for seven years, commented on what he and others had learned from David's life. He said that he taught David Religious Education in Year Seven and his memories of David then was of a quiet, rather reserved young man, who worked hard and rose to the challenge when things got tough. A sign of things to come he said! He then recollected how at the beginning of Year 11 David had gone into his office to announce that at the end of the year, after his GCSE's he was going to go on a Marine Conservation trip to the Philippines: to help sort out their marine conservation problems! I quote from John's memorial speech in The Hymerian 2006/7:

> It is clear from what you have just heard (from friends of David's who took part in the service) that David Hood made a huge impact on those with whom he came into contact.
>
> David was in all ways a splendid Hymers' student. He was very bright, he worked hard and was very successful, as his GCSE results showed. He was a great contributor; a superb athlete who did well at local, regional and national levels; he enjoyed his music and got

on well with other people in his quiet, undemonstrative way.

But when I remember David at school, I think of even more than all of that, because it was not just what he did but the character he displayed that makes him stand out. David made the impact he did on people not because he was loud and wanting to draw attention to himself. In fact, I remember a rather quiet boy when he was young, but he had a great sense of character and determination, and he developed an extraordinary gift of being able to sort out priorities, knowing what was important in life, and then doing the right thing with enthusiasm, commitment and with a smile.

When he was in Year 11, David came into my office to tell me about his planned diving trip to East Asia to help preserve coral. He spoke enthusiastically about protecting the environment, which he cared so much about; but with David, it was not just words - he was actually going to do something. Sadly, of course, it was on that trip that he first became so ill. And it was whilst he was ill that the true qualities of this remarkable young man became so apparent. When last summer (2006) he popped into my study again, in spite of all that he had been through and was still going through, his cheerful and positive approach, his deep faith in a God who loved him and his desire to share that with others, left me, for one, feeling very humble indeed.

I suppose the rather hackneyed phrase, "When the going gets tough, the tough get going" could have been invented for David Hood. Put David on an athletics field against powerful competition, and his response was to go for it, and his ability coupled with his determination made him one of the top competitors in the country; or inform him that the world's coral reefs are in danger and off David goes to sort it all out, or give him

AS level exams to do only last January, when he was not fit enough to do serious academic work, and he comes up with not only grade A's but 100% in his Mathematics paper; and tell David he has cancer and - well, you all know how he responded to that challenge. And it was these responses to the great challenges in his life, and his disarming honesty and desire to make the most of his life, not for himself but for the benefit of others - it was all these that inspired in all of us respect, affection and love. Of course, David's life was all too brief, but I have no doubts that in that short time he influenced more people positively and beneficially than many of us will manage if we live three, four, or five times as long as he did.

So I am sure that I can speak for the whole Hymers' community when I say that it has been a privilege to have known this fine young man. We extend to Sylvia, John and Tom and all those closest to David our sympathy, but also our thanks for allowing us to be part of David's life and for all that we have gained from that experience.

David leaves behind a gap that simply cannot be filled, but he also leaves memories that we shall cherish for as long as we live."

A fine and for me, his mum, a true and strengthening speech.

Ena Saltiel, a member of Beverley Baptist Church on a memory fish at the Service of Celebration wrote:

My special memory of David is whilst I had my leg in plaster. David was giving me advice on how to have a shower with a plastic bag on my leg! David was a very special young man. Whilst he was so ill himself he brought a smile and encouragement to others. It was a privilege to know him.

53

Another wrote simply "Courageous, motivational, inspirational, committed."

Hilary Hollingsworth, one of the staff at the Royal Orthopaedic Hospital in Birmingham, wrote:

> Fond memories of David, a unique and special person, who experienced and gave more in his short life, than most of us will do in a life time.
>
> His spirit and influence will live on through his family and friends and Coral Cay Conservation.

And from Peter Raines, founder of Coral Cay Conservation: "Loved by his Coral Cay Conservation family and friends".

And from Bilail, regarding David's faith:

> I remember how strong David was (we both have a strong belief in God) which I think sometimes would help us talk about his current health, however I was in continuous admiration of how emotionally strong and accepting he was of his illness. He always remained positive, even whilst we sat together and discussed how he wanted his funeral to play out.
>
> When I was told that David had passed, I remember I asked if I could come and say goodbye.
>
> I tried to keep everything together during David's funeral, but I struggled when his favourite poem (which then became my favourite poem) was read aloud, Footprints in the sand.

Recently, Phil Almond commented: "I miss David, his strength and light shone through every day. Everyone who came into contact with him was blessed."

Chapter 8
Video diaries

As I mentioned earlier, David made three videos about his experiences of cancer whilst on the ward at Jimmy's. He won a prize for the first video, in which he gives useful advice for people of any age having operations and chemotherapy for cancer (see earlier for the full transcript). Together with other video diaries, it was produced by Jimmy Teens to give to newly diagnosed patients.

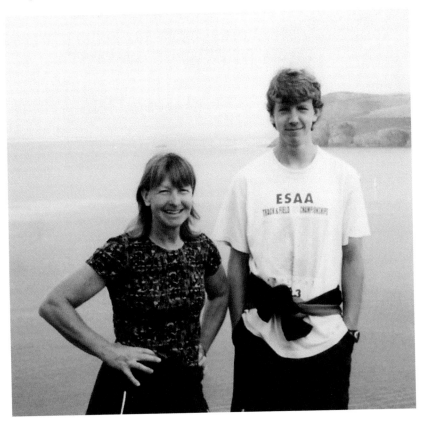

The second video focused on recovery after the leg operation and gluing of the lungs and looked at the importance of family, friends and a faith in keeping positive.

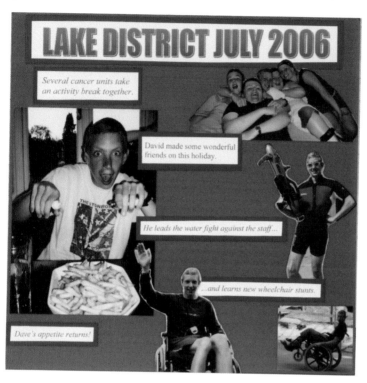

The third video, entitled "Find your sense of tumour" was shot at an international gathering of patients, friends and staff at Center Parcs. With the multi gold medalist, Marc Woods, three young people(David being one) aged 17, speak on how they have stayed positive. For David, it was through having the good support of family and friends, a faith (the Christian faith for him) and always having a focus, be it writing a booklet, making a video or fundraising - all of which he did on the ward.

Video 4 (Positivity) is a heavily edited copy of the BBC 6 O' clock news interview on May 16th 2007 in which David is being filmed the day after he has just been told he has about a month to live. Here again he talks to a specialist nurse, Sue Morgan, from Leeds about positivity and about what he has learned over nearly two years of treatment.

I found the unedited copy of this video at home last year. For the first fifteen minutes he talks about his favourite topic: Positivity. Then he asks Richard Bilton (special correspondent for the BBC and Tony Robinson (film crew) if he can be honest and bring them right up-to-date. He then tells them he was not well yesterday from internal bleeding and

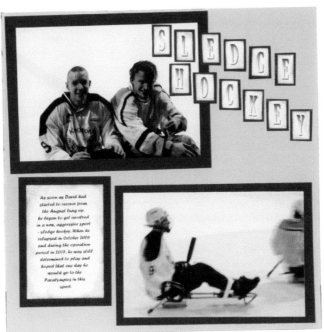

As soon as David had started to recover from the August lung op. he began to get involved in a new, aggressive sport - sledge hockey. When he relapsed in October 2006 and during the operation period in 2007, he was still determined to play and hoped that one day he would go to the Paralympics in this sport.

that he is only just digesting the news that he only has just been told that he has about four weeks to live! He then asks to be filmed explaining how he is facing the news of imminent death. We, courtesy of the BBC, have the moving and poignant discussions between David and Sue Morgan. I will explain a little about it later in the book.

57

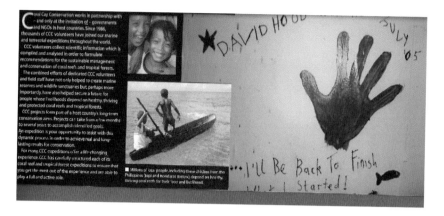

On the dive base wall – the Philippines. David left only one handprint not the usual two. He said he'd be back to finish what he started.

Three people who wrote comments on video 2 are Jacqui and Andy Lester and Dave Phillips:

"Dear David,
My name is also David and I found this website after I read an article on the BBC website in which you are mentioned. (It was the six o'clock news where he was referred to as 'the boy who moved the heart of the nation' when he was interviewed having just been told he had a month to live.) I did a Google search for your name as I wanted to find out more about you and how you were. Your films are very honest and moving. You seem to take all that has been thrown at you in your stride and even after just fifteen minutes of footage, your bravery and wisdom beyond your years shine through.

I am sat here on my computer in Wellington, New Zealand, writing this message to you. Although I should be working (I work at a company called Weta Digital who did all the special effects on Lord of the Rings) I felt it necessary to take time out to show my support. I hope you are feeling O.K. and still have your faith and family around to keep you positive. I wish you all the best and hope your days are happy and free from pain. I don't know you and you don't know me but your story has touched my heart and I pray for you."

58

Take care

David.

Also responding to video 2:

"Dear David

I too have just read about your fight with cancer on the BBC and wish to send you my warmest wishes and prayers at what must be a very challenging time. Your courage, your faith and your honesty are a true inspiration.

May you have strength to continue your battle and we shall pray not only for your healing but that your story can touch the lives of many suffering in silence."

Andy and Jacqui Lester.

Chapter 9
Positive responses throughout David's illness

There were many which are etched on my mind, but the ones numbered below are deeply etched in my mind.

1. Response from my phone calls with him during his time in the Philippines

    David was very anxious to find out what was hurting him so much in his leg, but he patiently took things in stages until we worked out together that there was something seriously wrong with his leg. He heeded my advice to focus away from the pain and to pray through it. Advice which set him in good stead for the rest of his life.

2. The first week back at home

    I was really impressed with David throughout the first week back at home in August 2005. He was in agony but seemed to take everything in his stride and made it a priority to see any friends not on holiday. It seemed a hassle to move him to take him and two friends to the Deep, but he was keen to go on an outing and have his camera 'baptised'. The Deep really rolled out the red carpet and made his visit memorable.

3. Three trips to the Royal Orthopaedic Hospital, Birmingham.

    David developed excellent relationships at the Royal Orthopaedic Hospital, especially with the consultant, Robert Grimer, and a member of the nursing staff called Hillary

Hollingsworth. He was a very poorly boy on his first visit and the thought was that he may not live the month out. However, he was determined to fight and fight he did.

On the second visit there he was put in the awful position of not knowing if the leg had been amputated or not. He coped remarkably well with this, focusing on mathematical computer problems to focus away from his anxiety.

On his third and final visit I accompanied him for a week's intensive physiotherapy. He worked so hard in the water and on land based machines to strengthen the few muscles that were left in the leg after the quads had been removed. Shortly afterwards he spent a good deal of time cycling. We bought him a bike and he was soon riding in and as soon as he was 17, being disabled, he was able to take driving lessons and soon had his own car.

4.   Sperm banking

I will never forget during his second week being hospitalised, chemotherapy was delayed in order to give David the opportunity of sperm banking, in case the treatment made him sterile. He was close to death, weak and uncomfortable. How he ever made it up several floors to a room where he could masturbate, I will never know. He gave a cheerful grin!

5.   Repeated lung collapses

These plagued David for the first three months of treatment. As the chemo went in and attacked the tumours of the lungs, holes would be ripped in the lungs causing David to fight for his breath until a skewer was put in and a chest drain. He often thought he was dying going through this procedure. He was so brave and positive.

61

6. Talks with Ian Lewis re: leg amputation

I will never forget one of David's consultations about being prepared to have his leg amputated! He was on chemo, being sick one end, diarrhoea the other end and carrying out a sensible conversation. Around this issue I will never forget his reaction to the thought of amputation: 'How will I walk in the Lakes with Tom?' he asked. Not how will I get to the Olympics now, but how will I have those lovely walks with my brother!

7. Lungs glued

Having an operation on the lungs to glue them to stop them collapsing was a real positive move and certainly a Hallelujah moment for Dave. Treatment seemed to be much simpler after that procedure.

8. Hymers' Christmas Ball 2005

After the leg operation and the gluing of the lungs, and after another round of chemo David was home for Christmas celebrations. Much to his delight he made it to the Hymers' Snow Ball.

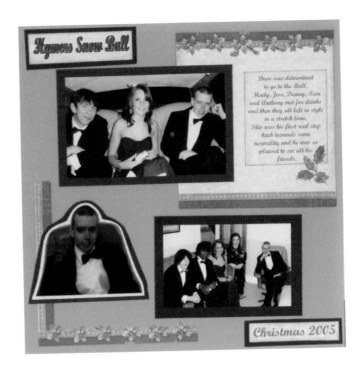

9   End of treatment, driving and Josh Cawley's
     Baptism

The period from New Year physio at Birmingham to
finishing chemo after Easter seemed to go by very

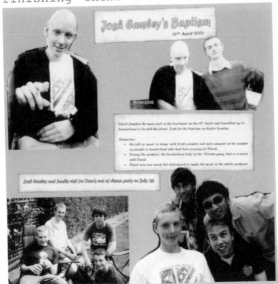

quickly. He positively learned to walk again, ride a bike and drive his very own car! The day after he finished chemo, we travelled up North with him to Sunderland, where he had arranged to go to his friend Josh's baptismal service.

He had met Josh on the Year 11 Florida trip and they discovered they both had a lot in common as Christians.

Reflecting on his memories of Hoody, Josh writes:

> Some people have a presence where others are simply drawn to them. On first meeting him, I remember wanting to be his friend. He had an amazing nature that brought people together. He did not show off: he simply communicated with everyone, making everyone feel at ease, as if we'd all known each other for years. In fact, we had all just met that day.
>
> Through Hoody's battle with cancer, our friendship supported each other through it. I believe we encouraged each other, pointed each other to God and helped each other see the bigger picture; I know that he did those things for me. Just like the day we met, his communication made me feel at ease, despite the difficult time. He was the one battling cancer, but he supported me: a true friend."

10. End of treatment Party

Josh and the rest of the Cawley family came down to Beverley to help us celebrate with an end of chemo party! It was such a joyous occasion. About two hundred gathered to be with us - friends from school, the Florida gang, friends from church and others. It was a great evening of music too with Tom Marrett's rock band and Peter Caswell on acoustic guitar and a good Ceilidh band. A memorable event, which is captured on David's second video.

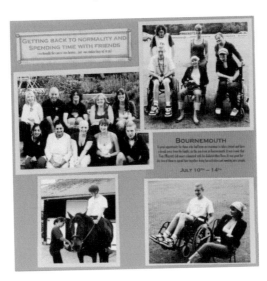

11. Ireland and chest X-ray

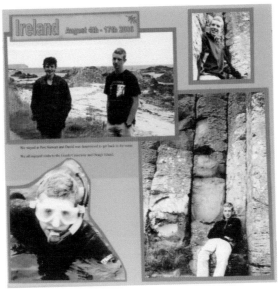

That summer we went for a well-deserved family holiday in Ireland - a week with the boys and a week for them to have time on their own in England with John and me spending another week together. Between the two weeks David had to have a chest x ray to show dead bits left on the lungs for an operation at the end of the summer.

12. The dreadful day it all came back...response to Ian Lewis and at school

This was a particularly dark day. After the lung operation in the summer, David and John went for what we thought was going to be a simple check-up. How wrong we were! And how things had been kept from us. I still marvel at David's responses on this day. Ian Lewis had to break the news that during the operation in the summer the surgeon failed to have his x ray with him! Apparently, it had gone to the wrong ward. Therefore he missed a new growth, which was now large and required an immediate operation and resumption of chemo. But the worst was still to come. David was told that he would not survive the return of the cancer and he might live just past his 18th in March! He could choose just to die naturally or have more operations and chemo to prolong his life. He opted for extension. He was then asked:

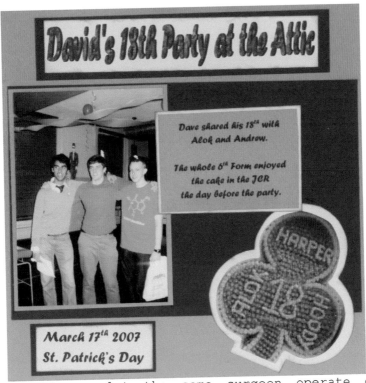

David's 18th Party at the Attic

Dave shared his 18th with Alok and Andrew.

The whole 6th Form enjoyed the cake in the JCR the day before the party.

HARPER 18

March 17th 2007
St. Patrick's Day

"Would you let the same surgeon operate on you again?" "Yes", was Dave's reply. "He won't make a mistake again". John and Dave were then told that he would never operate on a child under his care again and that Jimmy's would have an internal enquiry to find out what went wrong.

Dave then drove to Hymers to tell his friends and me, and, yes you've guessed it…to organise a party that night at our house.

I remember well the Deputy Head John Tinnion coming to my classroom door and asking me to go to the Head's office, where David was. I burst out crying when I heard the news and my 17 year-old son said, "I think I'd better drive you home, you're in no state to drive," and he did. That night John and I sat in the car in a lay-by and cried as Dave spent much needed time with his mates.

67

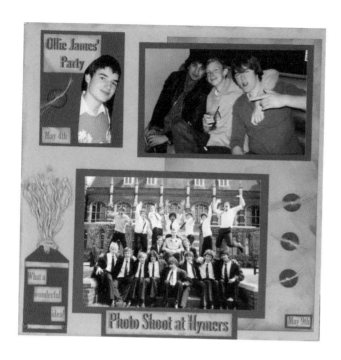

13 May 16 2007.interview by the BBC and Anthony's
    comment

On May 15 2007 David was told the cancer had spread
to all of his internal organs and that he had about
a month to live. He took the news so bravely. He had
internal bleeding and was struggling to eat. The
next day the BBC were filming on the unit and were
going to avoid David due to his tragic news.
However, somehow he managed to get chatting with the
film crew. For about fifteen minutes he avoids his
news and talks about positivity. He then asks Sue
Morgan, the nurse talking with him, if he could be
honest about his situation. I found the unedited
video last year. It is very moving and profound. It
makes me very proud of David, my son, as I watch and
listen. He explains that he is not afraid to die –
he had known God in his life and would be with him
through eternity. "I'm more concerned with how I am
going to die! If the tumours on the lungs cause
suffocation or drowning, that will not be nice." Sue

Morgan assures him that he will not suffer. He goes on to recall how traumatised he was by the death of another patient who was afraid to die. Elaborating, he says that he cannot think of anything worse than being afraid to die. You can almost see his brain working when he then starts thinking and joking of being dosed up with morphine, thrown out of a boat at sea, to be eaten by sharks! "I can't think of anything worse," Sue Morgan gasps.

"It might upset the food chain." David jokes.

He then goes on to talk about his funeral, "I want it to be full of music and extravagant."

He explained how he wanted it to be moving so that his wonderful friends and family could let all their emotions out and then get on with their lives. "You can't do anything when you're sad. And I don't want anyone to be sad."

"Do you think you will still be with your family?" Sue asks. "I will always be with my family." David replies. "But I like to be independent. There will be a big party in heaven and I will see all those who have died!"

I'm not looking forward to the wait for everyone else. This really moved me when I first watched the video. I don't know what to do with this video. It's very special.

Anthony Perera, a good friend of David's, accompanied him to the Find Your Sense of Tumour event at Center Parcs where Dave spoke so eloquently. Later on, he put pen to paper and recorded his thoughts and experiences with Dave:

> Dave had a vast knowledge on music. It was quite a central part of our friendship. We would always discuss music and he would always suggest artists to me. Two artists that I remember in particular were The Velvet Underground & David Bowie, who have ended up being major influences on my taste and pursuit of music. Imparting this knowledge of music and general discussion helped him get his mind off cancer during those days.

69

Of course, one of the more memorable times I spent with him was our time at Center Parcs. Dave was very comfortable here with a combination of friends old and new. This mixture of two worlds put him at ease and we enjoyed each other's company and friendship. One thing I still remember clearly was his fearlessness. He would not be scared to go around on his wheelchair doing various tricks and just going down hills as fast as he could. I, on the other hand, was understandably nervous every time he suggested doing these exercises. Dave was never angry about his situation. He was so many years more mature than we were. He was very clever and was interested in science as I was. He was a dogged and determined individual, un-phased and always looking ahead. I believe his strong faith played a large part in this. I am not a particularly religious person but Dave handed me the poem, 'Footprints in the Sand' which is a beautiful poem and one that I am very fond of. As his friends, we realised how important religion was to him and we would go to prayer meetings to show our support, even though some of us were not religious."

15. Back on a Coral reef in Tobago and reunion with Jan, the marine expert in the Philippines.

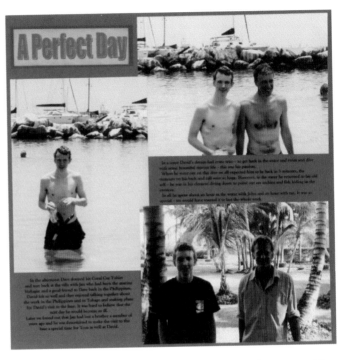

David lived the next four weeks of his life to the full. He went to as many 18th parties as he could before his dying wish 'to snorkel or dive on a Coral reef.'

He wanted to go back to the Philippines but it was too far and he was not well enough. So we booked a luxury holiday for the family in Tobago, where Coral Cay Conservation were also working. Finances for the trip came from Beverley Baptist Church, a charity called "Dreams Come True" and ourselves. Just the insurance was a thousand pounds as he was so close to death. We had a great but stressful time, with one bleed. You can see from the photo how happy he was to be on a coral reef again.

71

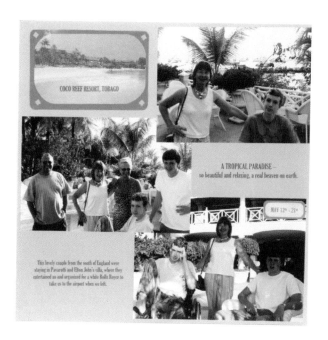

COCO REEF RESORT, TOBAGO

A TROPICAL PARADISE –
so beautiful and relaxing, a real heaven on earth.

MAY 12th - 21st

This lovely couple from the south of England were
staying in Pavarotti and Elton John's villa, where they
entertained us and organized for a white Rolls Royce to
take us to the airport when we left.

16   Final get together with his closest friends at
      Mady Stanley's home

After this with about one week to go he had a final
get together with his closest friends at Mady
Stanley's home. It was full of moving scenes –
laughter, long glances at friends etc and he was
clearly very weak.

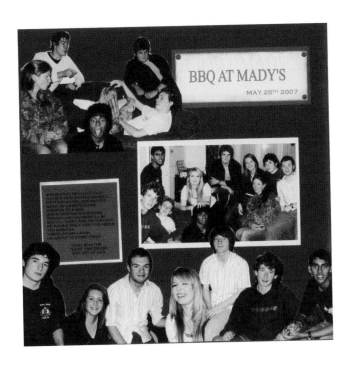

BBQ AT MADY'S
MAY 25TH 2007

17. A Glimpse of heaven

A day or so later, a strange but wonderful thing happened to Dave and me.

'The night in question I had got up from my bed to go to the loo and popped in to see how Dave was....

"It's beautiful, the music is beautiful...the balance, the harmony, it's beautiful, perfect. I wish you could be with me" Dave said.

"What music? Where are you David?" I asked

"It's beautiful", David replied.

"Are you in heaven?" I questioned. This seemed to be the right question.

"Yes, it's beautiful, I wish you could be here with me." David replied.

He then gave me a great big bear hug and said "I love you very much Mum"

"I love you very much too David," I replied.

He repeated "I wish you could be here with me" and then he lay down again.

It was a special moment for both of us.

Thursday May 31st 2007. A week before he died.

The next day he wanted to talk about what happened, it was as if heaven met earth! My friend Sue Banbury came round and went up to see Dave. She recalls:

> The final weeks of David's illness was the time in my life when more than any other I felt that the veil between heaven and earth was so thin that you could reach out your hand and touch it. There were so many people coming and going to visit him, and the home seemed so busy but at the same time there was a sense of awe and wonder, as if we were being allowed a fleeting view of eternal mysteries. When a couple of days before his passing David told me a little bit of his 'Glimpse of Heaven' it seemed to confirm all that I was feeling at that time - that indeed heaven was so close that it was all around us, just a breath away. I felt so privileged to have been able to share in even a small part of this with him and the family.

David's good friend Jonny Davies, who he had known since Hymers Junior School (and who is on the photo with David at the Deep when he was first so ill), wrote down his memories of David:

> I first met David, if I remember correctly, towards the end of Year 5. David was due to join my class in the place of another boy who was due to leave at the end of the year. David came in for a day to be shown around and Josh Duffield, a friend of mine, and me were asked to look after David and show him around while he was new. We soon became friends, and the rest, as they say, is history.
>
> David and I shared a real love of music, and in particular anything considered 'rock' in the loosest meaning of the word. One particular musical memory I remember clearly is going to see a Pink Floyd tribute band, Think Floyd, with David at Hull New Theatre. We both had a great time hearing the band play mostly better-known Pink Floyd songs, but they also played a couple of more obscure Syd

Barratt-era tracks, much to our delight. A lot of my friends will claim to be huge fans of music, but I remember fondly being able to discuss both the well-known and the obscure tracks, the stories behind the songs and the bands, and much more with Dave. The times I miss David the most now are often linked to music. For example, David was a huge Stone Roses fan, and when I went to see them in their first reunion gig at Heaton Park in Manchester in 2012, I couldn't help but think how much David would have enjoyed seeing one of his favourite bands reunited.

Even at his funeral, David left a nice musical surprise which makes me smile to this day. In the months before David's passing, he would sometimes talk about what song he would want playing at his funeral. Frank discussion like this was cathartic, for me at least, but he would usually settle on a sombre, downbeat song, most often 'Asleep' by The Smiths. At Dave's funeral, imagine my surprise when, having been completely prepared for a sad, poignant song to be played, the cheery, upbeat 'Good Day Sunshine' by The Beatles was played at the end of the ceremony. To this day, that song immediately brings back fond memories of David.

Another particularly fond memory of mine is a gathering we had at Madeline Stanley's house, a mutual friend, for a barbecue. Many of David's friends turned up. It was beautiful weather, and despite the fact that David was battling his illness at the time, I like to think that he had a great time too. There are a number of photos from the time which always make me smile and which I think sum up the mood of many of David's school friends at the time — it was hard to know what to do sometimes, but we tried our best to be there for David, and in doing so we had some great times.

The final week is pretty much a blur now, so many visitors, so many broken nights. Thankfully Dave had his close friends with him right near to the end.

Mady Stanley and Miriam Bennett were with him and about three hours before he died he sent them down to say it was time they should go. 'You'd better go then', I replied. No sooner had they shut the door then a congealed mass like a lump of liver came out of his mouth. Following this we seemed to be changing the bed every half hour with diarrhoea and then we noticed blood in what had seemed like poo. For the first time we called for a nurse to come. He didn't think it was signs of the end. John and I were not sure.

About midnight the nurse suggested we got some sleep and he went to be with Dave. Soon he was knocking on our door for John who went in and had a cuddle. I couldn't settle and went in to see David. I asked the nurse to go. He said he would stay downstairs. I was concerned about Dave's breathing so I sat with him holding his hand and praying. Another large burst of blood and poo came out of his back end and it stank! I ignored in and slowly watched David's breath disappear. It was so peaceful. I didn't know if he was dead or alive. He was so still. I prayed for half an hour with every ounce of faith that he would be raised from the dead. It was not to be.

I went and woke John. "I think he's gone." I said. We both held his hand and prayed and then went to fetch the nurse.

Those who die in Christ will live eternally. I tried to focus on this thought.

I was numb and felt as if I'd run twenty marathons. When I was writing this book I asked John how he felt at that moment. 'Numb' was his reply and feeling like he'd run a marathon.

We decided not to wake up Tom because the stench of death and mess surrounding David was so bad.

He finds it hard to talk about David, so I've never asked him how he felt. I do know that he would have like me to have woken him as David was passing away. I've explained that there wasn't time and I delayed getting his dad.

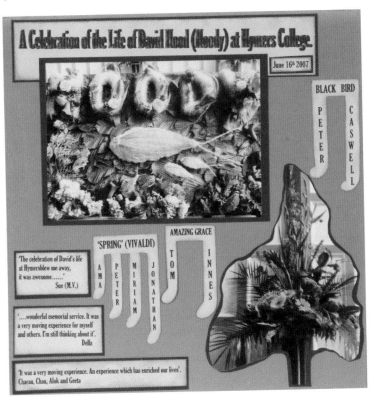

A Celebration of the Life of David Hood (Hoody) at Hymers College.

June 16th 2007

BLACK BIRD

PETER

CASWELL

'SPRING' (VIVALDI)

AMAZING GRACE

AMA   PETER   MIRIAM   JONATHAN   TOM   INNES

'The celebration of David's life at Hymers blew me away, it was awesome......'
Sue (M.V.)

'....wonderful memorial service. It was a very moving experience for myself and others. I'm still thinking about it'.
Della

'It was a very moving experience. An experience which has enriched our lives'.
Charan, Chan, Alok and Geeta

David's friends' were certainly there for him from the start of his time at Hymers, through the two years of such an awful illness and right up until three hours before he died, as I explained. And they were first rate! And they were there just hours after he died too, before even the undertakers had seen to the body.

I remember it well. It was a warm June morning and after having two doctors certify the death, we were sat out in the garden having a coffee. We had let Hymers know that David had passed away, as agreed, before we let anyone else know. This was so as not to interfere with Dave's friends' exams. So as they came out of the morning exams, the Head, David Elstone, gathered them together to break the news. Within an hour the first friend, Bilail Iredale arrived at our home with a gorgeous flower arrangement. I have the glass dish it came in in front of me in my dining room as I type! One of my best friends Adele, who is Irish then arrived and then the undertakers! What a gathering. Adele in good Irish tradition, asked to go and say goodbye to Dave. Which we were happy for her to do. Then Bilail, a boy of faith, asked if he could go and say goodbye. The protective teacher in me nearly said no, but the parent and 'friend' of all David's wonderful young friends who had lived through hell with us, said yes of course. Before anyone else arrived, the undertakers asked if they could just bung the back end of Dave and then added, you can keep him at home for a few days if you want. This seemed the right thing to do.

With his friends' help, David had written the Service of Celebration of his life and the Cremation Service. So I felt compelled to see that his wishes were carried out and Hymers College and Beverley Baptist Church were top of the class in helping me fulfil his wishes. There was lots of music and involvement of many of his friends. Some carried the coffin, some read, hundreds of others paid their respects in the usual way. It was an amazing service and a fitting send-off. How did we, as a family, feel you may well ask. I really can't say. Tom cried, John was quiet and I was as high as a kite! It was as if I was putting on an important school assembly, or nativity play, but not saying goodbye to my beloved son!

Chapter 10
The legacy of David's life

A tree in the North East

The students sponsored by Sunderland University, who had been on the Florida trip with David were a fantastic support to him during his treatment, and came and spoke at the celebration of David's life. Paul Jameson, the student liaison officer and Josh Cawley, one of the pupils gave an excellent PowerPoint presentation. After the service they contacted me to say that they had decided on a fitting memorial for David, bearing in mind his love of conservation and the environment: an oak tree.

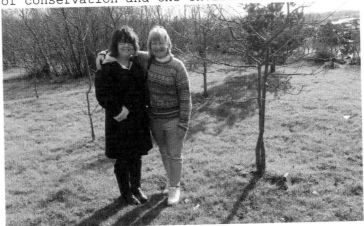

Josh Cawley's mum, Beth

It was to be planted in The Remembrance Garden at Herrington Country Park. A plaque was put against the tree: In loving memory of
David Hood
(Hoody)
17.3.89 - 7.6.07
"I feel good in a special way
I'm in love and it's a sunny day.
Good Day Sunshine!"
The Florida Crew 2005

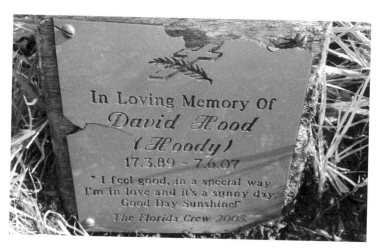

The family were very touched by this. David had chosen this Beatles song to be played at the end of the service of remembrance at Haltemprice Crematorium as the people came out and went to the service of celebration at Hymers.

Another lovely response was from a group of David's close friends. They decided to put their money together to buy a trophy for Hymers College. The trophy was donated with the specific instructions that it was to be presented each year at the school's Speech Day. This annual event was very academically focused and in contrast the trophy was to be presented to the pupil who made the greatest impact on the community at home or abroad. Each year since David's death we have been invited by the Head to the Speech Day to meet the new recipients of the trophy. This has kept us in touch with the school.

The Head of the Junior School had a large wooden bench made and on the top is carved David Hood - Pupil, sportsman, smashing lad. 1989-2007. A lovely gesture.

In memory of David, John and I decided to sponsor a child in the Philippines as close to where David was when he first became so poorly. Since 2007 we have sponsored John Bagado, who was fifteen this year. He is sponsored through Compassion UK and his education

80

and medical care are paid for. It is an excellent scheme.

In 2009 I met a young girl called Princes when I was travelling in the Philippines and I was very impressed with her maturity. Sadly she had lost her mother, brother and sister in a mudslide which had covered part of her village of Guinsaugon, killing all the children and teachers in the primary school there. In 2012 I managed to get in touch with her again and began some sponsorship to help her move towards some of her dreams in life - to live and work in the UK.

After David died I went straight back to school and to cut a long and painful story short, towards the end of the autumn term 2007 I was physically, mentally and emotionally exhausted. The message I was receiving from my doctor was that if I didn't stop pushing myself I would never recover. I was alarmed and stressed. After a couple of months of confusing deliberations, I ended my contract. The void that then hit me like a ton of bricks, floored me and nearly drove me mad. (I may write a book about that time as it came back to haunt me in ways no one could have anticipated.) Suffice to say I needed something to focus on. I was 53. Most of my close friends were still at work, as was John. I struggled greatly with this time and charity work kept my head above water. However, when in 2016 I had to finish Sport for Everyone, set up in memory of Dave, all the trauma came back to haunt me in the form of severe ruminations, causing bouts of depression.

Three thousand pounds from the Celebration of David's life went to form a memorial fund with Coral Cay Conservation (CCC). It was to target local young people in Tobago and the Philippines, teach them to dive and understand how to preserve the marine environment. I decided I would approach CCC and build a programme of a year abroad of voluntary work taking part in marine conservation and teaching sport and other subjects as the need arose. I thought this would 'finish off' things David had started, prove to be a fitting legacy and bring closure for me. John was still working full time, so I was on my own for the year.

So, at the age of 53 I set off, on my own, on a 'gap year': a little later than most people!

My first port of call from September 2008 until Christmas time was the beautiful island of Tobago, where we had taken Tom and David a few weeks before David died.

Here I worked voluntarily as an Education Officer. Primarily I concentrated on building relationships with schools and the local community and organised marine focused Education Days. One of my most memorable experiences here was spending an hour and a half free diving with a large pod of dolphins. They were great fun to be with.

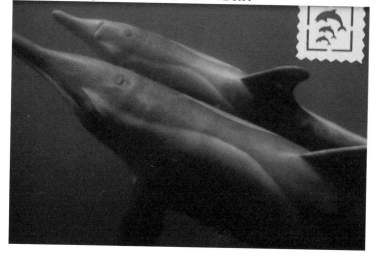

It was great to get home at Christmas and see everyone. I was positively buzzing. I couldn't seem to rest. I did a school assembly at Hymers, organised a large social event with a PowerPoint of the work in Tobago and saw loads of people. But I never really rested or set out clear plans for the next year. It was therefore, with some fear and trepidation that I boarded the plane to go East - this time, to the Philippines.

It was a long journey and I think I talked the whole way. Nothing new, many of my friends would say! However, behind the chatter there was a degree of anxiety as to what the next six months would bring.

When I arrived, late at night, Manila was a hive of activity. It was a noisy, bustling place that met me as I stepped out of the arrivals lounge and I was relieved to see a taxi driver with my name on his board waiting to greet me. He was very friendly and we chatted in broken English as he wound his way through busy streets of Manila. The hotel room was pleasant but I felt very vulnerable and alone. I barely slept as I was so concerned that I should not miss my next flight down to Tacloban. There I was met by CCC volunteers and driven to Napantao.

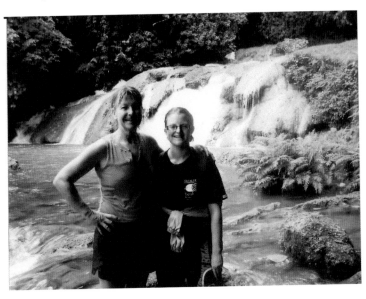

There were good times in Napantao, where I eventually arrived at the Coral Cay Conservation base, but there were very difficult and distressing times too.

I met beautiful people. My dream of seeing a playground Dave and I had helped fundraise for, was broken. That, coupled with having to prematurely leave the CCC base, plunged me into despair and depression. I will write more in another book.

I did enjoy diving and caving there. I also enjoyed meeting the people of Napantao and the survivors of the Guinsaugon mudslide. I was moved to tears as I saw David's handprint on the wall of the dilapidated base he had spent hours in agony at and my heart and soul cried as I heard how his screams had been heard a mile away and how when the locals had heard of his cancer, and the fact that at sixteen he was the youngest volunteer to visit, they were going to build a memorial to him. To me, the playground at the New Guinsaugon and memory of all the children lost as a mudslide covered their primary school was the memorial I wanted to see! I did all the planning for the playground and then, sadly, for a range of reasons, Justin would not release the funding I needed. I met with the mayor and the community leaders and organised all the paperwork necessary for planning permission but I never saw the playground finished. Appallingly, in my eyes, it was only just finished last year!

After the Philippines I went home for a short period and then John and I had a wonderful holiday in China, traveling by train, boat and bus from Beijing to Hong Kong. It was a fantastic holiday but I was not well. I suffered with what I now realise was depression during this time so didn't get as much out of the trip as John did. However, I don't regard this as part of David's 'legacy'. The next trip, however, most certainly was and I am very pleased with what I managed to achieve there.

I had planned to finish my year's trip with a month in the Maldives, followed by a month in Africa, but things developed rather differently.

Setting off on my own again after being with John seemed quite daunting. In retrospect I was in depression and experiencing extreme anxiety. At the time I didn't really know what was wrong with me or how to deal with these emotions. (See my next book for more detail).

84

Thankfully I was met by a good friend in Male and she seemed to understand the grief I was experiencing better than I did. She had organised a gradual introduction to voluntary teaching and I soon settled into a programme of work in a range of schools in the capital, Male and then further afield to the non-touristy inhabited islands.

I eventually ended up at Dharavandoo where the plan was to stay for a week and alongside a sports teaching programme, teach some PSHE (Personal, Social and Health Education). On the first day I had some free time and it was easy on this small island to walk to a beach in any direction. I headed for the nearest beach and was disgusted with the sight that met my eyes - rubbish everywhere. The beach was covered with all kinds of rubbish and literally hundreds of plastic water bottles. Naively I had expected something akin to a tourist island I had visited. It was no better when I went snorkelling. There were tampons, disposable nappies, plastic bags and the like tangled round or dangling from the coral. It was disgusting to me! What would David think? I thought. Over the next few days I decided that I should do something positive, on the marine conservation side of things, in memory of him. So, alongside coaching sport and visiting other islands and eventually bringing staff to Dharavandoo from other islands to a sports conference, I put together a massive island clean-up plan. In order to fulfil the plan I had to radically change my travel itinerary and carve out more time in the Maldives. To do this I cancelled my flight to Kenya and organised a trip to India (out of the country) so as to extend my visa. Again, I suffered a bad bout of depression whilst on my own at a beautiful beach hotel/spa in Kerela.

Once back in the Maldives and focused on the conservation plan I was fine. Whilst I was away, Aamaal had arranged a week's conservation trip with a group of Male students and some keen conservationists. It was an excellent week. The starting and finishing point proved to bring my plan up a gear and add to its feasibility. I was introduced to the beautiful island of Soneva Fushi [es@soneva.com.] and its wonderful owners - Sonu and Eva. How their wonderfully generous offer came about, I really don't know. Suffice to say they heard of my plans for Dharavandoo and offered for me to have a break on their luxury island before starting the project. Even more amazingly they offered to support me in the project!

So, I went from travelling around with a group of students and wadding through the mangroves and the like to living in the lap of luxury. My beach bungalow had three showers - one inside, one on the terrace and one on the beach. The island had its own recycling unit and a magnificent observatory. If I'd been paying, it cost around £1,000 per night to stay there! I was staying for free! The evening meal cost around £150, but I was given the option of eating for free in the staff restaurant. An option I jumped at.

During the day I cycled round the island, snorkelled, planned the Dharavandoo project with staff and dived. It was Manta Ray season and I have fantastic memories of one particular dive. I was clinging to a rock, poised with my underwater camera mesmerised as about twenty to thirty Manta Rays swirled and glided above me. A truly epic moment. A magnificent sight. We would then climb into to the most luxurious, padded up deck dive boat and sip champagne and nibble melon and grapes as the sun warmed us and we relived the dive. Opulent living. The time there certainly gave me a rest, and the opportunity to plan the reef and beach clean-up at Dharavandoo.

The week soon passed, goodbyes and thanks exchanged and I was ferried by speed boat to Daravandhoo, where I was to stay for the next couple of weeks. Instead of staying with a family this time, I was staying in an empty house on the school site, right next door to a very active mosque. Yes, you've guessed it - woken at the crack of dawn by the call to Morning Prayer and then four more sessions throughout the day. I soon learned to tell the time by this routine. On parallel tracks I coached sport in the school and planned a community conservation project to be done in memory of David.

Two weeks of work culminated in a grand community reef and beach clean-up which was actively supported by the staff of Soneva Fushi. Basically, the children were occupied all day on a carousel of sports, art and musical activities and only had two half hour slots of litter picking. The adults on the other had collected the sofas, filing cabinets and the like from the beach, and general rubbish, and gathered it all in a huge mountain on the harbour side. Boats of divers collected rubbish from the reef. A fun, productive time was had by all. Some had said I would only get a handful of people to help with such a project. Amazingly, 350 out of a community of 500 got involved. I was chuffed.

The task of disposing of all the rubbish then met me. Again Soneva Fushi came to the rescue and it was arranged that for as long as was necessary their waste barge would call and take all there rubbish to the disposal island near Male. David would have been impressed with this whole project. It was televised by a local company but I haven't seen the recording. However, I still have fond, proud memories.

It was tough being back in England and job wise nothing seemed to develop that inspired me. So, in 2010 I decided to do a year of fundraising for the Teenage Cancer Trust (TCT) as a kind of thanks for all we had experienced on a TCT unit and to help other families going through what we had been through. My friends were fantastic at supporting the events that I did, roughly every three months - a sports event at the leisure centre, a strawberries and cream garden party at the Stanley's (Mady's parents) and a Barn Dance. In total around £4,000 was raised. It was hard work, partly because I was in and out of depression: something I had never experienced before I lost Dave.

In comparison, £36,000 was raised in one day with Viking fm. Basically, they organised a phone in 'Auction of Promises' and I was in the office all day helping with the phone calls and other activities. Sandwiched between the auction and records, and played throughout the day, was an interview they had recorded with me as to what difference the TCT made to a hospital unit and what difference a four bed unit at Cottingham would make to young people diagnosed in Hull and the East Riding of Yorkshire. It was a fantastic day and I was amazed at the amount raised.

Around the same time, in 2010, I had an idea to start a family sports evening called Sport for Everyone. The concept was to go against the tide of segregated groups and activities and to have an all age, multi-activity evening aiming to develop social, emotional, spiritual and physical skills. I didn't want the evening to be solely a 'Church' event but I was keen for it to bring together people from all the churches in the area and none: For it to attract and serve people of faith and none and folk from all backgrounds. I am pleased that it has evolved into a lovely, well respected group ranging in age from about three to 82! We met fortnightly or monthly for seven years up to 2016, when, due to highs and lows of depression, the time seemed right to call it a day and the resources were given to help continue inter-church work, open to anyone.

This is an amazing legacy to an amazing young man.

We take nothing from this world, it's what we leave that matters. I will leave you with the words of Mady, one of David's closest girl friends. She sent a card saying:

Dear Sylvia, John and Tom
I really just wanted to write this letter to explain and simply say what an honour and incredible experience I've had, growing up and having Hoody by my side!

I started to get to know Hoody on the 923 school bus and journeys from home and school. Me, him and Tom would sit and talk, being the last ones off the bus. Then I remember during GCSEs, me and my brother taking the train home with Hoody on warm summer evenings. And of course I remember his fundraising night for the Philippines, that was truly the first time I recognised what a great guy he is. So when I cam back from Canada and heard the news, I simply felt shocked, I just couldn't imagine someone in our year, our friend was ill and all we wanted to do was to be there for him in any way we could. But, from the start it was when we visited him in hospital I assuredly knew I visited him never out of pity, but because I genuinely, thoroughly, totally and absolutely love Hoody's, no matter his state, as he's just so much fun to be with. I have always loved how different aspects of his personality fuse to create, …well, Hoody! He's genuine, courageous, kind, practical, amazing, wonderful human being.

I've learned a lot from Hoody, things that have and will affect for the better, the way I want to lead my life. I learned fundamentally from him that life is what you make it: Hoody presented a project to Hull University and was able to venture to Florida, Hoody actively raised money for the Philippines and went to the Philippines. I learned that being proactive makes people around be proactive too. From him I learned that in the darkest moments, light and hope shines the most brightly. I really learned to appreciate the seemingly tinny things that can brighten up a whole life! I remember being on the phone to Hoody when he knew he was terminal and him just describing to me how sunny and beautiful the day was, I love that he always sees the positive in everything as that's simply how I would and will aim to live my life like as well. I've also promised to learn how to dive, not just learn but become good as I really want to explore the world that Hoody is so passionate about. He is securely In my heart, as are the whole of the Hood family! I really would love to have a long standing friendship with you all, only if you'd want it of course!

And, of course, I'd just dearly want to thankyou for how humbling and hospitable you've always been, letting us into your home and allowing us all to be as involved as we have. The whole experience with it's painful, negative aspects has also been an honour, being able to spend time with the whole Hood family.

Sorry this is so long, I know you've had heaps of cards delivered to you!
Lots of love.
Mady.

The singing in David's 'Glimpse of Heaven' moved David in the depths of his being. It moved me too. It's the closest I have been to God in my life. The song goes on. This may be the end of my book, but it is not the end of the story ...and I guess, the story never ends.

Sylvia xxx

31233021R00056

Printed in Poland
by Amazon Fulfillment
Poland Sp. z o.o., Wrocław